DELTA
MEDICINE

DELTA
MEDICINE

Natural Therapies
for the Five Functions
of Cellular Health

Yann Rougier, M.D.

Translated by Kiki Anderson

Healing Arts Press
Rochester, Vermont • Toronto, Canada

Healing Arts Press
One Park Street
Rochester, Vermont 05767
www.HealingArtsPress.com

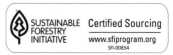

Healing Arts Press is a division of Inner Traditions International

Originally published in French under the title *Se programmer pour guérir: La Delta-médecine: de nouvelles réponses pratiques face au cancer*
First U.S. edition published in 2012 by Healing Arts Press

Note to the reader: *This book is intended as an informational guide. The remedies, approaches, and techniques described herein are meant to supplement, and not to be a substitute for, professional medical care or treatment. They should not be used to treat a serious ailment without prior consultation with a qualified health care professional.*

Library of Congress Cataloging-in-Publication Data
Rougier, Yann.
 [Se programmer pour guérir English]
 Delta medicine : natural therapies for the five functions of cellular health / Yann Rougier.
— 1st U.S. ed.
  p. cm.
 Includes bibliographical references and index.
 ISBN 978-1-59477-464-5 (pbk.) — ISBN 978-1-59477-685-4 (e-book)
 1. Cancer—Alternative treatment. 2. Cancer—Diet therapy. 3. Detoxification (Health) 4. Cancer—Psychosomatic aspects. I. Title.
 RC271.A62R6813 2012
 616.99'40654—dc23
                                                              2012009903
Printed and bound in the United States by Lake Book Manufacturing, Inc.
The text stock is SFI certified. The Sustainable Forestry Initiative® program promotes sustainable forest management.

10   9   8   7   6   5   4   3   2   1

Text design and layout by Virginia Scott Bowman
This book was typeset in Garamond Premier Pro with Trajan Pro, Gill Sans, and Myriad Pro used as display typefaces
Illustrations by Cécile Mazur

I dedicate this book to each one of you, sick or well; to all the health care professionals who find these suggestions of interest; to their patients as a way to open a new space for dialogue; to all those who suffer; to those close to them as a way to open a new space for understanding. To those of you who no longer want to suffer, who want to understand more, understand that a part of all healing is contained within each of our actions and each of our thoughts. Learn to replace ancient fears with a new consciousness, a new confidence, and then a new certainty: All of us have within us the means to program ourselves to heal.

And this book is to Josette Rousselet-Blanc, an exceptional person, a brave heart with a destiny stronger than illness. She has dedicated her professional life to women and women's health and her personal work to providing information, offering hope, and listening, through her organization, Association Étincelle. This book is based on transcriptions from a series of conferences held within the Étincelle organization (www.etincelle.asso.fr); the conferences and workshops were organized in order to help, support, and better inform patients.

CONTENTS

FOREWORD

As Dr. Yann Rougier pertinently reminds us, the great Plato offered a holistic vision of the health of human beings. I like the adjective *holistic* because it evokes plenitude, with its Greek root *holos,* as well as the sacred, with the word *holy.* This forms a whole, or, to use the author's geometry, a magic triangle, a delta, in order to preserve our health.

I confess that at the beginning of my medical practice, which focuses on the malignant afflictions of adults as well as children, I was rooted in scientific proof. It was difficult for me to accept that cancer, the uncontrolled growth of unhealthy tissues that sometimes caused death and was implacably physical, visible, and aggressive, could be influenced by psychological factors. Multiple thoughts, mental images, emotions, feelings—what did the mind have to do with the malignant mutation of our cells? It didn't seem to me that psychologists had the appropriate tools to offer any convincing proof.

But as luck would have it, the agnostic oncologist that I once was would one day meet a great psychiatrist who specialized in a comprehensive, holistic approach to the personality of patients. Pierre Marty was recognized by his peers for the originality of his thinking and the quality of results obtained with his collaborators in the field of physical afflictions. This hotheaded researcher with a tumultuous spirit and a lively intelligence created the Psychosomatic School of Paris. It was he who helped me take seriously a domain that I had scorned up until then. Because we were both "passionate pragmatists," we took the risk of running double-blind tests to ensure the validity of our results. In other words, neither the patient nor the specialist knew the diagnosis at the time of the evaluation. The results of this study proved that interactions between the body and the mind were indeed real. I now recognize the place it has earned within this discipline.

Yann Rougier offers us a very interesting book, clearly the fruit of his life's work and personal research. He offers an approach to well-being and healthy living on several levels, based on good sense and balance, that is easy to carry out by taking "little Delta steps." The Delta symbol is a good choice because it presents an image of harmonious interaction that dovetails with the overall vision of the author.

We live in a world that is permeated with stress and pollution. Well-being on a daily basis is an objective for all of us, whether we are in good health or sick. Yann Rougier's approach is centered on illness prevention. But it also offers important insights for patients, complementing their medical care.

I wish the author much success with this book.

PROFESSOR CLAUDE JASMIN, M.D.

Claude Jasmin, M.D., is a professor of oncology, hematology, and immunology at the Medical College of University of Paris XI, chairman of the board of oncogeriatry at the Institut National du Cancer (National Institute of Cancer), and president of the Institut du Cancer et d'Immunogénétique (Institute of Cancer and Immunogenetics).

ACKNOWLEDGMENTS

To Professor Claude Jasmin, the living spirit of the masters. Your interest is greatly appreciated and your foreword is a thrill and an honor for *Delta Medicine*. Thank you for your advice, your warmth, and your motivation to expand a field that you yourself initiated through your many collaborations with hospitals.

To Jon Graham, my editors Jamaica Burns Griffin and Diana Drew, Cynthia Fowles, and the entire team at Healing Arts Press, for their confidence, trust, patience, and professionalism.

To Marie Borrel and Caroline Pajany, for listening, for their patience, and for their motivating creativity.

To Marc de Smedt, for a whole life in the service of others.

To Alejandro Jodorowsky, for his deep and generous knowledge about the ties that unite the heart, the body, and the mind.

To Marianne Costa, a symbolic hyphen between my thoughts and my pen!

To my wife, Valérie, and my sons, Loïc and Jauffrey, the coauthors of this book: I created the text, they made the spaces between the words come to life.

To Marylène and Jean-Pierre Pouysségur, Pascale S., Nathalie B., and Philippe M., for proofreading with honesty and kind but clear comments, often as valuable as the ideas themselves.

INTRODUCTION

Modern medicine has reached a point where it cannot guarantee good health unless you work in conjunction with your physician. . . . Our power to prevent and heal illness is far greater than most of us realize.
DENNIS T. JAFFE, *HEALING FROM WITHIN*

The therapeutic goal of Delta Medicine's five tools for health, developed in this book, can be summarized in one single sentence: Put the medicine of the body at the service of the medicine of man.

What is this *medicine of the body* that, for centuries, preceded manmade medicine? It's what we see at work each day when wounds heal, then disappear; when bones mend; or when thousands of bacteria are neutralized by fever and then evacuated. Since the dawn of the human species, the primary healer has been the body itself, even if we take it for granted and trivialize these "biological miracles" that occur daily.

Sometimes, however, the blow is too strong, the wound too deep, the bacteria too prevalent, or the body too contaminated or weakened. Then modern medicine takes over. But in applying these medical or surgical tools of healing, we must not forget, or, worse, undermine our own tools of healing that are connected to the life of each of our cells.

The life of a cell is infinitely rich and complex, but it rests on five key functions: a cell breathes, eats, eliminates waste, communicates with other cells (thanks to the nervous and hormonal systems), and, finally, creates, expresses, and controls emotions (thanks to a rich form of communication and collaboration between neurons). The five tools of the Delta Medicine program have been developed to rebalance and reinforce these five factors of cellular health.

Of all the challenges encountered during a lifetime, one of the most important is making choices that let all our processes of healing—and self-healing—manifest and reinforce one another. Take the well-informed advice of your family doctor and that of all the specialists she recommends: this is the first and most indispensable option when facing any illness. Read this book attentively, and try the healing tools with serious intention: this is the second option that I offer you.

These two options are not at all contradictory. Rather, they are fully compatible. They are the two complementary paths to healing and renewal, with a full awareness of being whole in body, mind, and emotions.

This book is for both those who are sick and those who are well. The latter will be able to use the effective tools of prevention, while the former, confronted with the urgency of an illness, will focus on the aids to healing.

This is why those who are sick and wish to quickly begin practicing the Delta Medicine techniques can refer directly to the exercises marked with a triangle, the geometric figure that symbolizes the capital letter *Delta* in Greek (Δ), without first reading the entire book. In addition, each chapter concludes with a summary of Key Points—a useful recap to come back to and a valuable resource for those with limited time.

Our therapeutic approach reflects wisdom several thousand years old that has gained renewed attention today. As Plato noted more than twenty centuries ago, "The greatest mistake in the treatment of the human body is that physicians are ignorant of the whole; for the part can never be well unless the whole is well." With the dawn of the third millennium this insight—both lucid and wonderful—joins the most recent applications and the most promising syntheses from neurosciences (see appendix 4), traditional mind-body medicine, and modern psychoneuroimmunology.*

Delta Medicine is a proven response to one of the greatest scientific challenges of the twenty-first century: lifestyle diseases, also known as diseases of civilization, most prominently, cancer. These chronic pathologies are one direct consequence of our frenzied march toward progress and a science that is superb but too often lacking a human dimension.

The complete Delta Medicine program brings together five tools for health, designed to return strength, hope, and, above all, a human shape to healing. These practical tools were created and then brought together to respond to the five major internal imbalances directly connected to our way of life. Without our realizing it, these organic imbalances can construct, or generate, within us, day after day, the symptoms that precede major lifestyle diseases: cancers, autoimmune diseases, viral diseases, and the multiple degenerative diseases.

The five Delta techniques are aimed at helping you better manage your breathing, your diet, the process of cellular cleansing, and stress. They will also aid you in harmoniously managing your emotional turmoil and quieting your inner fears.

In short, Delta Medicine is a program designed to awaken all your inner forces of healing, your full potential to heal yourself. This program cannot promise you an immediate return to health, but, based on my several decades of experience and reflection, I can assure you of progressive and long-lasting well-being.

Please note that I've included a glossary at the back of the book, where I define terms that might be unfamiliar to you. If you come across a term that you don't understand, check the glossary, which begins on page 247.

---

*Psychoneuroimmunology is a branch of neurosciences started by American and Canadian schools in the 1980s (from the work of Dr. O. Carl Simonton and Dr. Bernie Siegel), then largely adopted by universities the world over. It focuses on the influence of emotions and thoughts on our immune, hormonal, and nervous systems.

This book is the best synthesis that I can offer from thirty years of research and thorough observation of the laws that rule our internal equilibrium.

When an author writes a book, he does so in his own words. Those who read it rewrite the book by integrating the spaces that separate the words into their reading. If they color these white spaces with the nuances of their thinking and personality, the book then becomes theirs.

I would like you to make this book your own. Then, together, we can open the door that leads to the path of your healing. But you and you alone will turn the knob and step through the doorway. You and you alone will take on the challenge of healing and health. Make the decision now. I wish you a safe journey on the way to your renewal.

THE BASIS
OF DELTA MEDICINE

*For most of our existence as a species, we have not had
doctors, whether conventional, alternative, or otherwise.
The survival of the species alone implies the existence of a
healing system.*

DR. ANDREW WEIL, *SPONTANEOUS HEALING*

BECOME THE AGENT OF YOUR HEALING

Delta Medicine is a program of awakening all our healing energies.

If you are holding this book in your hands, it is because illness
concerns you. Perhaps you have contracted one of these lifestyle illnesses, such as cancer, whose diagnosis in Western societies continues to
increase. Perhaps someone close to you is faced with this type of illness.
Or perhaps you want to do all that you can so you won't have to suffer
this kind of serious medical hardship.

Cancers, as well as autoimmune and degenerative diseases, have
multiple causes. In other words, numerous factors, human and otherwise, figure in their onset and development, among them genetics,
nutrition, viruses or bacteria, inflammations, various kinds of pollution, stress, and emotional pressures. Western medicine, also known as

allopathic medicine, applies symptomatic treatments to patients with these types of illnesses. The effectiveness of these treatments is confirmed by research. But alongside these treatments, which are sometimes intense and often accompanied by painful side effects, it is always possible for you to take action yourself. It is always possible for you to take control of certain physical, nutritional, mental, and psychological realities of your life to help your body and your mind better unravel the numerous threads that form the illness that has developed within you.

This is what Delta Medicine offers—a range of simple techniques that are easy to integrate into your daily life, to help you find your way back to a healthy life as quickly as possible.

DELTA MEDICINE: A NEW THERAPEUTIC SPACE

Ever since the second half of the twentieth century the amazing discovery of antibiotics has allowed us to fight major infectious epidemics very effectively. Yet the Western world has seen other types of pathologies emerge that are more difficult to diagnose and treat: degenerative diseases, autoimmune diseases, and, above all, different forms of cancer. Along with chronic fatigue syndrome, multiple allergies, and troubles with depression, these form the vast group of illnesses called lifestyle diseases. Today these illnesses have begun to affect developing countries as well, where their growth is often exponential, with cancer at the top of the list.

These diseases are not due to a particularly virulent infectious agent or known organic injury. Rather, they are linked to the overall biological state of the patient. We often refer to the overall biological state of the patient as the *terrain*. When a person is ill, we also talk about the *weakness* of the terrain on immunological, hormonal, digestive, and even psychological and emotional levels. In addition to how an imbalanced terrain figures in illness, we also consider the impact of heredity, pollution, and viral infections.

Lifestyle diseases stem from a variety of attacks on the system, or metabolic, immune, neurohormonal, psychoemotional imbalances. All these factors are implicated to varying degrees, depending on the case. This is why these illnesses are characterized as multifactorial. Western medicine combats these diseases with molecular therapeutics that are often effective but sometimes too symptom-based (that is, too monofactorial) and more likely to provoke serious side effects without promoting a lasting recovery.

Keep in mind that these treatments (chemotherapy, hormone therapy, immunotherapy, radiation therapy) are often indispensable to addressing these diseases. You cannot seriously treat cancer without contemporary Western medical guidance and testing. But patients who do so are not always completely satisfied with their treatment—physically or psychologically. It is within this context that Delta Medicine can help. How? By offering simple and natural health-promoting tools that complement contemporary medical treatments and optimize their effects, while revitalizing our healing energies so that we may recover. It is this combination of therapeutic synergies that allows us to rapidly improve our well-being, recuperate, and find our way back to health.

DELTA: THE LITTLE SOMETHING THAT CHANGES EVERYTHING

Delta Medicine is based, in part, on a fundamental psychosociological statement from which it takes its name. Delta is a Greek letter used in mathematics, physics, and biology. In everyday language, it means a "little something." But attentive sociomedical observation has proved for centuries that human beings are extremely reluctant to make big changes, whether on a physical, a psychological, or a spiritual level. We are very attached to our daily habits and big upheavals profoundly disturb us. However, we can integrate major changes in a timely manner when an emergency forces us to do so. And the emergency triggered by the diagnosis of a serious disease (especially cancer) generates profound anxiety, which can then give us the energy to abruptly change our habits. But this kind of attitude also generates intense, repeated stress that, in the end, erodes our willpower, no matter how determined we may be. New habits and all-or-nothing changes are so difficult to integrate into our daily life that, in the long run, we rarely realize their beneficial effects. And the stress, frustration, and social and family pressures engendered by these externally imposed new behaviors tend to undermine the beneficial effects that we do see. In short, these drastic changes lead to a form of social alienation whose impact on our psychological and emotional equilibrium is disastrous: we no longer eat like everyone else, we don't share the same schedules and rhythms of life, and so on.

On the other hand, in order for any long-lasting changes to occur it is essential for us to make these changes in a moderate way. Step by step, as the saying goes. To that we would add, Delta change by Delta change. Delta Medicine calls for us to integrate small changes into our daily life that are simple and progressive, that don't demand significant changes in our lifestyle, and that won't disrupt our medical, familial, and social relationships. The result will not be any less rapid or effective; it will only be less abrupt. And since these Delta changes don't cause frustration or stress, the positive results we obtain will last much longer. This will allow us to build within ourself, day by day, a true program of awakening all our healing forces.

DELTA MEDICINE AND CONVENTIONAL MEDICINE

This health care program is not meant to challenge or undermine any conventional medical theory. The tools of Delta Medicine come directly from medical techniques used in hospitals and found to be effective in scientific research performed in universities. But sometimes these techniques are neglected, either because the medical profession brands them as too incidental or not offering results rapidly enough (for example, nutritional techniques, phytotherapy procedures, oligotherapy, and enzyme therapy), or because, although deemed effective, they demand an investment of time and human involvement that is too extensive (for instance, the autogenic training of Dr. Johannes Heinrich Schultz, guided mental imagery, sophrology, symbolic mind-body medicine, and Jungian imagery).

Adopting Delta Medicine techniques does not create the awkwardness we sometimes feel when we hide from our doctor our decision to pursue complementary techniques that are not always well known or well regarded by contemporary Western medicine. At the same time, Delta Medicine may lessen disagreeable side effects from traditional treatments. Therefore, it acts in positive synergy with all the techniques sanctioned by contemporary Western medicine.

Finally, Delta Medicine's five tools for health are dedicated to the development and reinforcement of all the processes of our body's own healing. We must never lose sight of the fact that the world's first medicine is the natural responses of a sick body. These are the processes of the body's healing. Whether it is a wound, contact with an infectious agent, a twist, or a sprain, the first response is the medicine of the body. When that is overwhelmed—either because the wound is too serious or the infectious agent is too powerful—Western medicine must then take over.

Our program is grounded in a set of three core therapeutic principles designed to promote bodily health: healthy nutrition; anti-stress and anti-fatigue breathing techniques; and simple detoxification of the body. There are two other, more personalized tools as well, to better manage the flow of thoughts and the negative impact of certain emotions.

Delta Medicine presents these tools for healing by connecting them in a dynamic way, in an overarching vision that reinforces the effectiveness of each technique. The sum of Delta Medicine's "little things" can unblock a "big thing" for you, promoting overall health and well-being. It begins with your active participation in your healing program.

MODIFY YOUR LIFE GENTLY

We now know that all lifestyle diseases—cancers, degenerative diseases (neurological, articular [diseases of the joints]), autoimmune diseases (multiple sclerosis, lupus)—stem from multiple factors. We must try to pinpoint the factors that contribute to the weakening of the biological terrain, leading to a more profound imbalance: disease. A major factor is always cited, wrongly, as if it were a curse: genetics. However, as long as a condition is not congenital, genetics does not underlie it. While all health issues that arise and develop are based on an individual's genetic weak points, this transgenerational weakness, or predisposition, is first and foremost abruptly triggered by our living conditions and habits.

These are the five principal factors involved in the weakening of our terrain of health and the construction of all our chronic illnesses, particularly those that concern us here—various types of cancer, as well as degenerative, viral, and autoimmune diseases.

- Factor 1: Bad control of breathing (amplitude, rhythm)
- Factor 2: Nutritional imbalances and deficiencies
- Factor 3: Pollution (notably, nutritional and atmospheric)
- Factor 4: Excess stress and nervous tension
- Factor 5: Management of emotions (principally, the resentment/ guilt pair and feelings associated with them)

Some clinical studies (official but very specialized; see appendix 4) have shown the importance of each of these, as much in the onset of diseases (their *construction*) as in the recovery from them (their *deconstruction*). Along with standard treatments and accredited procedures (chemotherapy, radiation therapy, corticosteroids, and anti-inflammatory drugs prescribed long term), numerous doctors who work in hospitals have verified the importance of a healthy diet, an optimal intake of certain unsaturated fatty acids and antioxidants (without uselessly overdosing on them, which, paradoxically, may actually aggravate the disease rather than alleviating symptoms), a detoxification cure and draining of certain vital organs (liver, kidneys, digestive tract), and regular psychoemotional self-evaluation (autogenic training pioneered by Dr. Schultz, sophrology) or mind-body techniques (conscious walking, the Feldenkrais method, chanting, breath control).

FOR THOSE WITH SERIOUS ILLNESSES AND THOSE IN GOOD SHAPE

All the health-promoting behaviors that Delta Medicine offers concern each one of us, even outside the scope of a diagnosed serious disease. The techniques are equally useful for those who are well and wish to remain so as long as possible. Delta Medicine therefore offers a true base of prevention.

We are all born to live, and to live fully. When illness and disease weave their web within us (and we will see that, unintentionally, we often maintain this state of health for years through our bad habits), we must replace "death reflexes"* with "life reflexes." This is what each of the program's tools offers.

I know from experience that we can favorably influence the course of an illness, no matter how serious it may be, by eating better, breathing better, keeping stress to a minimum, and managing emotions that are too strong or date from too far back yet continue to overwhelm our present life.

As you progress, and as your well-being improves and you place more confidence in these Delta techniques, you will be able to look in to deeper explanations, if you wish to, and dive in to the more detailed questions and responses found at the end of the book (see appendix 2).

---

*Please excuse this term. I use it to indicate that certain behaviors can truly send you progressively into the brutal world of degenerative illness, beyond your genetic predispositions and beyond your destiny. All of us must realize this and react; we all have the means to do so within our reach.

TOWARD A CONVERGENT MEDICINE

One last clarification: All the Delta Medicine techniques are "natural" in the sense that they use the therapeutic resources of the body—organic, nutritional, psychological, emotional—without appealing to chemical treatments as a first resort. But they are not classified as "alternative" medicine. Numerous patients with serious illnesses seek help via different therapeutic routes (and some positive results have been achieved with these alternative modalities), but approaches such as acupuncture, osteopathy, homeopathy, fasting, the mono diet, Ericksonian hypnosis, and so on are largely absent from hospitals. I would nevertheless emphasize that doctors who are open to these practices have often come to modify their perception of the doctor-patient relationship, to the patient's benefit. They offer their patients more listening time, more detailed questioning regarding their daily habits, and a more in-depth consideration of their peripheral imbalances (that is, imbalances in nutrition, thoughts, and emotions).

Problems arise when what is called alternative medicine is placed in opposition to contemporary Western medicine. Even more troubling is that while complementary practices have their virtues, the fact that they are often termed *alternative* keeps them from acting in synergy with conventional medicine. The tension this creates (more in some countries than others) is detrimental to the patient, who rarely dares to tell the treating doctor about these personal initiatives. And when the patient does venture to do so, the response is at best an awkward silence, sometimes politely expressed doubts, or at worst strong criticism. Those who practice alternative medicine, some of whom aren't doctors, may give advice beyond their competence with regard to the conventional treatment protocol. Unfortunately, this undermines the credibility of the positive results of their technique. This terrible waste could be easily avoided with legislation that is more tolerant but also better regulated and stricter—as is the case in Germany, Japan, and Canada.

Even more regrettable, this misunderstanding between conventional and alternative medicine always works to the detriment of the patient.

Delta Medicine is not meant to be an "alternative" to Western practice or hospital treatments but rather to be convergent with it (to use a geometric but elegant image). I don't claim that this is the ideal way to heal any disease. Rather, I have created an approach that is medical, ethical, tested, and internally coherent. Through this approach, which realigns different therapeutic influences that are carefully selected, and makes them convergent, we can reinforce the effectiveness of all conventional therapies, sometimes diminishing the side effects, and, in the end, favorably influencing the overall process of healing over the long term.

Nevertheless, our approach also introduces some original ideas. First of all, Delta Medicine sheds new light on the way disease constructs itself within us. This means that we can attempt to deconstruct it if we understand the underlying processes and thereby reverse them or, more precisely, rebalance them (see the following chapter).

Delta Medicine also distinguishes itself from contemporary medicine by incorporating techniques from mind-body medicine, an approach that associates directed thoughts, emotional assessments, and symbolic acts within a specific protocol that takes into account recent applications from the field of neuroscience (see appendix 3).

I must reiterate that these tools for health are all meant to enhance conventional medical treatment. While doctors might view these tools as ancillary to your treatment, they won't consider them doubtful or dangerous for your state of health.

All the therapeutic forces can then work together in full transparency and synergy, supporting your healing energies.

Key Points

✢ The second half of the twentieth century saw an exponential increase in lifestyle diseases. These are principally illnesses with a nonmicrobial origin: degenerative diseases, autoimmune diseases, viral diseases, and, above all, cancer.

✦ Their point in common: These are illnesses with multiple causes. This means that they develop as a result of imbalances that are metabolic, nutritional, environmental, psychological, and/or emotional.

✦ The treatments offered in hospitals in response to these types of diseases (chemotherapy, hormone therapy, immunotherapy, radiation therapy) are all indispensable, but are not always sufficient or satisfying on a humane level.

✦ Delta Medicine offers simple techniques that join together with conventional treatments to improve the well-being of patients and facilitate their return to health.

✦ Delta is a letter from the Greek alphabet used in all fundamental sciences to designate the first step of a transformation, or a small variation. Delta Medicine consists of a group of small behavior changes, capable of having major effects on our health and quality of life when practiced in synergy. Human beings don't like making big changes; big changes generate stress, frustration, and social alienation. That's why this program offers small changes that work in tandem with one another for enhanced, long-lasting, therapeutic effectiveness.

✦ Delta Medicine does not work in opposition to contemporary Western medicine and hospital treatments; the two are complementary. Delta Medicine stimulates and awakens the healing mechanisms that constitute our very first medicine—the body's medicine.

✦ Delta Medicine offers five targeted tools (breathing, nutrition, detoxification, relaxation, and management of emotions) that respond to the five principal causes of our organic imbalances (bad respiratory habits, poor nutrition, pollution, stress, and negative emotions).

✦ Delta Medicine is also very effective for people in good health who are interested in actively preventing lifestyle diseases.

THE CONSTRUCTION AND DECONSTRUCTION OF ILLNESS

Our behavior, feelings, stress levels, relationships, conflicts, and beliefs contribute to our overall susceptibility to disease. . . . By improving these dimensions of ourselves over which we have control, we can maximize our well-being and our ability to resist illness.

DENNIS T. JAFFE, *HEALING FROM WITHIN*

The set of techniques presented in this book have been created to accompany you on the path to healing and well-being. We view this progression as possible because disease is slowly constructed within our organism due to five negative or destabilizing factors (bad respiratory habits, poor nutrition, pollution, stress, and negative emotions) and can therefore often be deconstructed by means of rebalancing techniques in conjunction with traditional treatments and the usual therapeutic procedures.

In the same way that negative influences have led to a gradual imbalance in the body, other positive influences (health strategies that are consciously applied) will counter these processes and work toward balance and a harmonious reprogramming of your metabolism. Therefore, it's important to first determine what these silent, hidden mechanisms are—the five destabilizing factors that prepare the terrain for the majority of degenerative diseases and illnesses (see page 10).

WE ARE BORN HEALTHY

Life should be considered an incredible miracle. We generally associate it with a newborn's first appearance, his or her first breath and cries. Sometimes the sense of wonder begins before that, when you can feel the small being move inside the mother's belly. Yet the true miracle of life begins much earlier, at the invisible (and therefore less emotional) moment when the "winning" spermatozoid meets the "consenting" ovum. This race for life includes millions of candidates for one sole "elected," and seems to me even more magical than birth because it is at the moment of this encounter that two genetic codes agree to mix and give birth to the first cell of a new human being, a person with his or her own looks, character, thoughts, and emotions. What a miracle!

This primordial cell already contains a nearly complete "instruction manual" for the construction of the body. Cell by cell, biological phase by biological phase, over the course of this incredible program of construction, of plasticity and cellular evolution, the embryo will become a fetus, then a newborn. This baby will become a child, then an adolescent. And the adult will age and eventually become elderly. This vital process is made unique not only by the particular content of the initial mix but also by internal and external influences (our famous five factors) that play such an important role in the way the program of construction unfolds.

The question then arises as to what these forces are, the energy deep within, and the great internal and external influences that preside over the unfolding of this program we call life.

The newborn's first act of life in the world is that first inhale, that first primordial breath, that first cry. Then the hands and mouth reach for the mother's breast in search of food. This small being has become a bit more autonomous: he can breathe and metabolize food. The first two essential programs of life are in place. It's the same for each cell of the body: cellular breathing and nutrition allow it to exist, then set up all the phases of development.

- The nervous system commands the body, both consciously and unconsciously (the voluntary and autonomic nervous systems).
- The immune system defends the body from all aggressors, with all the nuances of the different populations of white blood cells.
- The combination of all the organic and nervous functions allows for the development of the senses, thought, memory, and emotions and the emergence of a distinctive personality. Little by little a being builds itself this way, brought up under parental influences and integrated into society by way of identification and confrontation with others.
- Finally, the sexual personality appears. This mixes all these energies in a more or less positive, harmonious way, signaling adulthood, or the emergence of the complete human. (As an aside, let us point out that new research reveals that more and more nuances characterize this ideal chronology of personality development. Sexual identity appears earlier and earlier, and is less and less structured and complete.)

THE CHALLENGE OF GENETICS

The vast majority of us enter this world in good health. This is the case for 99.3 percent of the population. The remaining 0.7 percent are unfortunately born with genetic illnesses or diseases that are more or less serious. The latter case occurs when the genetic mix giving birth to the first cell is incomplete, or "too complete," which creates from the very first weeks of life (sometimes even before) more or less serious disorders that appear with a group of characteristic symptoms. Among the most familiar of these are Down syndrome and cystic fibrosis. In addition, cases of cancer in very young children (from birth to seven years old) may require psychological interventions that involve parents and others close to the child in specialized therapeutic work in addition to medical treatment. These specific diseases largely fall outside the scope of this book.

Delta Medicine addresses, first and foremost, the countless people who were basically born in good health.* Our different metabolisms are well coordinated (breathing, nutrition, immune system, nervous and hormonal functions, emotional ebbs and flows); they function in a harmonious manner, balanced in terms of our initial genetic mix.

At the outset of our life force there is a fusion between two parental imprints that gives birth to our genetic identity. This is our first, and actual, moment of birth. The laws that govern this sharing of two parental contributions are not fully known, although genetic research over the past few decades has allowed us to uncover many of them. The genetic makeup that constructs and guides our life still guards some of its mystery. Similarly, although genetic biomedicine is a very promising field, it remains under the control of the laws of nature, which are a lot more complex and less predictable than simple mathematical formulas applied to genetic sequences via computers. Thus, when one single gene is deficient in one of the chromosomes, we might think that repairing it will suffice, or replacing it with a healthy gene could resolve the problem. This sometimes works within the context of an experiment using plants or primitive animals (cell and virus cultures). But the closer we come to the human species, the more complicated the process becomes. We encounter compensation genes that disturb or counteract the actions of the new gene, for example. It's as if the new gene were

---

*While Delta Medicine doesn't directly address severe genetic disorders, it can still offer both mental and physical support to the parents of a young patient—and others close to the child—who are confronted with the weighty emotional task of caring for that sick child.

taken for an intruder by the organism, even though it's the right gene in the right place. So the genetic challenge of the twenty-first century isn't solely a matter of bioinformatics. It isn't just about the decoding, sequencing, and retranscribing intended to map the genetic system and its infinite subtleties. This genetic challenge is definitely biomolecular, biohormonal, and bioimmune.

OUR BIG LIFE BOOK

We all possess a "life book" in which our base biological terrain—that is, our genetic heritage—is written in detail. But this book contains several chapters. The first concerns the making of the embryo. The second relates to the baby's arrival in the world and the start of the respiratory and digestive functions. The third deals with the growth of the baby as well as the development of its functions and vital systems. Then comes the chapter on adolescence, with its hormonal adventures, followed by the chapters on adulthood, and eventually old age.

Yet in all life books there exists without exception a special chapter titled "Organic Weak Points," where there appears, in the smallest of details, the specific weaknesses that, for the most part, affected our parents, grandparents, and great-grandparents. Some of these weaknesses may diminish from generation to generation. This is truly a blessing for those who benefit from this natural effect of compensation. But other weaknesses become more potent and form our personal weak points for the rest of our lives. These can have an impact on any of the organs, functions, tissues, or parts of the body. They can affect the breasts, the digestive tract, the prostate, the bones, the heart, the joints, and so forth.

Popular wisdom states that ethnic mixing produces stronger individuals. This is scientifically true. By mixing ethnic groups the risk of reinforcing the imprints of close genetic weaknesses, susceptible to becoming potent, diminishes. For example, the inhabitants of Western countries suffer from circulatory problems more frequently than the

Japanese, who, for their part, are prone to joint problems. An individual having a European father and a Japanese mother therefore runs less risk of developing one or the other of these two weaknesses, because the genetic fingerprints of the two parents are so different. A child born to such a couple will probably possess a life book containing a chapter of weak points that is smaller than that of either parent.

This leads us directly to a very important point that is necessary for you to understand and remember if you want to change your relationship to disease: the chapter on weak points in our genetic book will only be "read" and applied by our bodies during moments of great metabolic imbalance, or great physical or mental fatigue. The markings of our genetic weaknesses are nothing but an imprint of a potential disease, a predisposition to a disease that may or may not develop. A possible pathology may figure in your life book, but it is not inscribed in your organic body now, nor in the more or less predictable unfolding of your future. Even if it is perfectly visible in your genetic analyses, nothing obliges you to express it at any given moment of your life (unless, of course, it is a congenital disease, in which case it is apparent at birth). Therefore, if we can say yes to prevention without hesitation, we must absolutely say no to fatalism.

One essential question must then be asked: What makes a genetic weakness morph into a manifest, or "declared," disease? What characterizes this key moment when you tip over from being a person in good health to being a sick person? Delta Medicine defines this point of equilibrium between the two extremes, or this point of imbalance or transition, as the Delta Point. On one side is complete health; on the other, fully declared disease. By exploring in detail the metabolic components and organic characteristics surrounding this Delta Point, you will understand why we develop certain illnesses. On top of our already stressed and polluted life contexts, our daily missteps and repeated imbalances can provoke, little by little, a weakening or upsetting of our controlling organs, opening the way for the expression of our genetic weaknesses.

THE STEPS OF DEVELOPMENT

This is how chronic degenerative disease is constructed within us, slowly, progressively. It passes through several stages. First of all a person goes from perfect health to discomfort and uneasiness (chronic fatigue; physical and mental uneasiness; trouble sleeping; fibromyalgia; subclinical, or minor, depression). Then all this sickness takes shape and is distilled until it expresses itself as a very real disease that includes all the symptoms that coalesce into a diagnosis. In the same way that a human organism is built from one initial cell programmed to grow in to a human being, the disease is built on a cellular terrain, but in this case different negative factors interact. Some of these factors are genetic, others stem from the environment (physical, mental, or emotional). Daily life hygiene also plays a role (superficial breathing, nutritional imbalances, air and water pollution, excess stress, unhealthy emotions, negative and belittling thoughts). Even life events may figure in the development of illness (including bereavement, major losses, abandonments, sacrifices).

THE DECISIVE IMPACT OF DAILY BEHAVIOR

In our life book the "Weak Points" chapter may refer to numerous genetic imprints. And when, in addition to the varieties of pollution in our environment, repeated nutritional, respiratory, nervous, or emotional imbalances end up compromising the immune system, the disease will tend to take hold first at the level of one of the organs referenced in this chapter. (Here I refer to chronic degenerative diseases that don't have a direct correlation to external, direct, aggressive causes or pollutions, such as tobacco or asbestos.) Depending on how we live on a daily basis, how we breathe, eat, take care of our body and our neurohormonal system, how we respond and adapt to stress and manage our emotions, we will be led to express them via our hidden weaknesses. Disease is then declared.

A practical example: Some people are carriers of the genetic marker

HLA-B27, generally linked to rheumatoid arthritis, a chronic, degenerative, autoimmune disease that affects the joints of the body by way of inflammatory attacks. It is a painful, sometimes debilitating, and mentally exhausting disease. Some carriers of this gene develop the disease and others don't, depending on external factors essentially related to lifestyle. But that's not all. People who aren't carriers of this predisposing gene can develop rheumatoid arthritis if they accumulate certain imbalances through how they live. Hence the statement that a "genetic inscription" of a disease does not absolutely condemn you to develop this pathology over the course of your life. Likewise, the absence of a genetic inscription doesn't totally keep you from the risk of developing it. What is essential is not this genetic predisposition, which you cannot control. On the contrary, what is essential is the voluntary equilibrium that you can and must establish for the health of your biological terrain.

This is precisely the idea behind Delta Medicine: it strives to bring back the equilibrium impulse in your biological systems. And this whether you carry predisposing genes or not. It is in this sense that Delta Medicine helps you retrain and reprogram your body as well as your neurohormonal system, your breathing, your eating habits, and your emotions. It's also what makes it a true medicine of prevention, strengthening your biological terrain when you practice the techniques, even if you aren't sick.

OUR LIFE BALANCE AND THE DELTA POINT

Our body possesses a memory of the healthy state in which most of us arrived in the world. It will maintain this state at whatever cost, for as long as possible, because, as we noted earlier, fundamentally our body is programmed to heal itself.

Imagine a life balance: the pan on the left holds this memory of good health while the pan on the right is weighed down by the weak points found in that chapter in our life book and by our imbalances and daily aggressors, along with pollution.

This balance leans spontaneously toward the side of good health, because that's the pan that is naturally heavier at birth. But pressures and life errors progressively accumulate on the other pan. During an initial period (which may prove to last very long), the healthy side remains heavier. It oscillates depending on the accumulation of imbalances on the other side, but without ever passing the point of equilibrium. The body remains in overall good health.

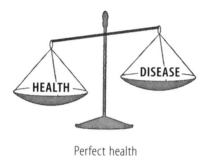

Perfect health

In fact, our body can support substantial imbalances, depending on the individual. Nutritional overload, nervous exhaustion, and emotional shock—in each case, as long as the healthy side of the balance remains heavier, we can withstand it. We can overeat from time to time without suffering from indigestion, and even if we don't dress warmly enough, we'll barely get a sore throat. A violent emotional shock may affect us for a long time without necessarily making us depressed. The damage will remain in the realm of acute, common diseases that Western medicine knows how to control.

But by weighing down the sick side, all these imbalances accumulate and end up making the scale tip sharply. At first, the two sides are equally weighted. The body enters into a predisease zone, and the symptoms, up to this point acute, become recurrent, then chronic. The body can no longer easily manage the ordinary, day-to-day imbalances. The physical, psychological, and emotional bad habits and missteps begin to leave their mark, and medicine no longer treats them as effectively. Five-day colds become flus that last weeks. Your mood remains dark. You feel out of sorts, less and less well, less resistant to illness and less resilient once you get sick. The first signs of disease appear: trouble sleeping, depression, multiple aches and pains, and persistent, inexplicable fatigue. These problems rapidly become chronic.

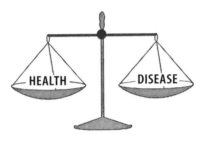

The Delta Point

If we consider these first signs as warnings, and we adjust our attitudes and behaviors without delay, the scale can rapidly tilt back to the side of health. If we do not, the healthy side will have more and more difficulty compensating for the weight on the sick side. Then comes the moment when the scale tips toward the side supporting the weight of our genetic predispositions and our accumulated bad habits. The Delta Point has been crossed. The scale leans inexorably to the side of chronic or degenerative disease.

Once we surpass this point of equilibrium (even slightly), this Delta Point, everything becomes more complicated. In the first stage, disease is declared. It is visible, clearly identifiable, and classifiable by way of its symptoms. The scale continues to oscillate, the person feels better or worse, depending on the day, but these oscillations no longer lean to the good side, the healthy side, for any length of time. Molecular medicine (that is, stronger medication or chemotherapy) delivers responses that have less of an impact on diseases of this type. Moreover, at this stage, *healing* is talked about less and less and only *remission* is discussed. This means that the profound metabolic imbalances underlying the illness are no longer under control.

Between these two extremes—perfect health and declared disease—

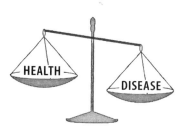

Chronic or degenerative illness

the oscillations around the Delta Point represent the sounding of an alarm. This zone of basic ill-being is like a flashing red light announcing a possible illness. It is an important warning that we must never ignore. This is the zone of ill-being in the twenty-first century, in all its forms. It's the zone of the *chronic,* of fatigue that rest will not ease, of depression lacking identifiable sources, of allergies and inflammations, of the viral, of the degenerative, of the idiopathic (meaning that we don't know the origin of the symptoms, so we treat these symptoms one by one without having an overall view of the illness). It is a zone that deserves a book of its own to describe, explore, and explain.

REPROGRAMMING THE DELTA ZONE

Once you cross the Delta Point, you then move over to the side of disease. At this juncture some people respond by improving their way of life by eating better, doing a bit of exercise, getting more rest, and keeping stress at a minimum. But these efforts, even if sustained, do not necessarily offer visible results within several weeks, or even several months. Discouraged, sick people then tell themselves that it's too late, that such simple acts would be ineffective in their situation.

This is a grave error! Don't forget that it often takes years of excess and bad habits to make the scale lean to the side of illness. By this logic, it will take time before your efforts succeed at making the scale tilt back toward the healthy side, once again crossing the Delta Point. Nevertheless, the good news is that the path back to health is traveled much more rapidly than the path to illness. Whereas it took years or even decades to go from health to illness, it takes only a few weeks or months for you to feel the first effects of your new healthy behaviors (provided, that is, that your imbalances have not led to the destruction of key organs). Keep in mind that your motivation must be clear and your efforts sustained. Sustained effort and perseverance are the keys that make all the Delta techniques work at full capacity.

The bad habits that weigh down the sick side of our life scale are numerous and varied. Some we all recognize: nowadays everyone knows that food that is high in saturated fat, too salty, or too sugary isn't good for our health, just as we know that an excess of stress is bad for the nervous system and smoking is bad for our lungs and our heart. Others are harder to discern: for example, most people aren't aware that breathing in a halted, broken way with the wrong rhythm tips the scale to the illness side. We'll also discuss contaminated food, lack of rest, violent psychological aggressors, emotional pollution, bad mental hygiene, and so on.

Delta Medicine focuses entirely on one goal: crossing back over the Delta Point. This is why the Delta techniques will accompany you daily, at first, on your path toward feeling better. Delta Medicine's governing principle is to send several messages of equilibrium each day to your main organic systems (digestive, respiratory, nervous, emotional, immune, hormonal) in order to reinvigorate them, promote their coordination, and make them weigh down heavily on the healthy side of the scale. Overall lifestyle correction will lead to a permanent, improved state of health. Once the bad habits that have led to the expression of genetic weaknesses and disease are corrected, the process can be reversed long term.

Another advantage, and a major one in my opinion: Once you have actively and responsibly participated in your own healing, you will be able to remain the central player in your well-being on a permanent basis. Your body is no longer an anonymous terrain of biological actions that is the exclusive province of doctors. The courage that this personal work requires will help protect you against the fear of relapse that often haunts patients after a serious illness. Knowing that you have control over your own well-being—and being able to support, help, and optimize your organic healing functions and your psychological and emotional equilibrium—constitutes an effective shield against the insidious anxiety of relapse. A vague sense of anxiety can eat away at the spirits of "cured" patients to the point of once again weakening their overall terrain and placing it in danger of relapse.

CONFRONTING FEAR

The fear of relapse is often a matter of residual anxiety, the tail of this comet that we call serious illness. It forms a persistent shadow that follows the fear provoked by the announcement of the disease. This may create a cataclysmic reaction. The patient feels overcome by a double whammy—that of injustice (Why me?) and that of the unknown (the disease thrusts the patient into a morbid reality for which he feels utterly unprepared).

Patients don't readily understand why their body has betrayed them so harshly. And, most often, doctors don't explain how the patients' (involuntary) actions contributed to the construction and development of the disorder that has brutally moved them from the side of well-being to the side of illness. This medical silence is usually well intended: doctors fear they'll add the weight of useless guilt to the already heavy burden shouldered by their patients. But there's a vast chasm between guilt (or the term I prefer—*involuntary participation*) and awareness, just as there is a chasm between responsibility and assuming responsibility. A precise but benevolent explanation emerges when we assume responsibility, thus allowing us to react effectively. Feeling guilty only gets in the way of finding practical solutions, and the situation then remains hopeless. This undermines the goal of returning to health and can even lead to depression. Assuming responsibility can prove to be a positive and constructive step—when it is done in conjunction with gaining a better understanding of the body and its mechanisms—one that allows patients to maintain their health and sustain the process of healing.

As long we don't know and don't understand the impact certain behaviors can have on our health, there is no reason to avoid them. On the other hand, when we discover how these behaviors weigh down the bad side of the balance, little by little, we can identify and replace them with health-promoting behaviors. Then, by taking the necessary measures to gently modify certain daily attitudes and activities, we can support our doctor's efforts to return us to health.

In this way Delta Medicine's active awareness of responsibility allows for a more direct collaboration between patient and doctor. Remember: we are born healthy. If a disease has progressively taken root within us, it is often because of processes that we must learn about in order to limit their deleterious effects. It would be absurd to feel guilty about not knowing how to breathe correctly, eat in a healthy way, and manage our thoughts and emotions. We live in a time when information about these areas is not a major concern. When we do hear about healthy lifestyle choices, it's often presented in excessive and contradictory ways, and therefore seems useless. You can find more than seventeen thousand diets, two million links to nutrition sites, and three thousand psychotherapeutic techniques on the Internet. So much disorganized information in the end will only confuse and misinform.

Because we must face our situation, we must seize the only opportunity that illness offers: it can make us interested in what is going on inside us and place us behind the scenes, closer to our cellular, organic, mental, and emotional life. This is how it provides us with the weapons that will help us fight more effectively, in conjunction with the most appropriate medical treatments and in close collaboration with the medical profession.

Words are nothing but words. We all do the best we can when faced with new information—even if it's positive—to digest it and then integrate it into our life. But whatever our strengths and our weaknesses may be, it is always easier to fight against an enemy like illness with an overall understanding of our biological mechanisms than to tackle it with vague fears and exhausting uncertainties.

Once you have digested and integrated this essential information and you understand what is taking place inside your body and mind, you will be able to participate more actively in your own healing. You'll not only be the agent of this healing, together with your medical team (who will remain the coordinator of your treatments), you'll become the owner of this healthy vitality. No one ever will be able to take this from you. This is your property for life!

Key Points

↣ We are all born in good health (except in certain rare cases of grave genetic diseases), and our body retains in its memory this imprint of good health.

↣ The moment the maternal ovum and the paternal spermatozoid meet gives birth to our genetic life book, which contains our organic strong points and weak points; strong points + weak points = individual biological terrain.

↣ Our genetic weak points may not express themselves during our entire life. They will only do so if we accumulate the five factors of imbalance targeting the way we (1) breathe, (2) eat, (3) eliminate toxins and internal pollution, (4) manage our thoughts and stress, and (5) manage our emotions.

↣ Our state of health can be viewed as a balance: on one side is the good health we received at birth; on the other, all the imbalances—innate and acquired—that lead us to illness.

↣ When the bad influences accumulate on the sick side of our life balance to the point that they become heavier than the good influences on the healthy side, disease is declared. It then expresses itself through our genetic weak points.

↣ In the same way that disease is constructed within us, we must try to deconstruct it by adding weight to the healthy side of our life scale.

↣ The five therapeutic tools of Delta Medicine allow us to add weight little by little to the healthy side so that we can reverse the movement of the scale.

↣ Before leaning to the bad side, our life balance must cross over a point of equilibrium, the Delta Point. Our body then alerts us by way of symptoms of chronic ill-being: fatigue, nervous tension, trouble sleeping, digestive difficulties, and so on. Sometimes the practical measures of Delta Medicine can prevent disease before it is declared by returning the life balance to the side of health (that is, before it has passed the Delta Point).

→ When you pass the Delta Point, these same health-promoting behaviors can accompany medical treatments and reinforce the natural processes of healing in order to return you more rapidly to a state of health.

→ Becoming conscious of the power of this mechanism allows you to be the agent of your healthy vitality. This also protects you from the fear of relapse, and this is essential for long-lasting well-being.

UNDERSTAND BETTER
IN ORDER
TO HEAL BETTER

Treating is explaining. Healing is understanding.
DR. JOSEPH MURPHY, *THE POWER*
OF YOUR SUBCONSCIOUS MIND

"More than 99 percent of us are born healthy and yet die early or suffer from premature disabilities due to an unbalanced life and environment. The important progress will come when each person accepts the responsibility of his or her own health. This calls for a change in lifestyle for the majority of us," explains John Knowles, former president of the Rockefeller Foundation.

The five techniques of Delta Medicine that we just covered and that we will reinforce through practice in the following chapters focus on the improvement of our breathing, nutritional habits, and systems of detoxification as well as a better management of stress, our thoughts, and our emotions. These are not radically new therapeutic targets. Some hospitals, notably in Canada, Belgium, and Germany, have already integrated many of the techniques presented in this book into their treatment protocols. But let's not forget that it is the synergistic and coordinated approach of Delta Medicine that makes all the difference.

AN INDISPENSABLE COLLABORATION

For more than a decade numerous complementary therapies have appeared in several fields of treatment, particularly for cancer. Some hospitals offer patients targeted nutritional programs, psychological support, and emotional management protocols. But let us be clear: no induction therapy (a first step in treating cancer), whether nutritional, psychological, or psychoemotional, claims to directly cure cancer. Beyond the efforts of neuroscience, numerous techniques aimed at psychotherapeutic support and mind-body integration have for many years helped patients better manage the emotional impact of their disease.

But, strangely, only in the case of certain serious neurodegenerative diseases, such as Alzheimer's, have we seen a closer collaboration between chemotherapy and psychobehavioral (and therefore psychoemotional) therapies.

For the moment, within the vast domain of organic diseases, attention remains focused above all on the cellular and organic imprints and impacts, possibly genetic, sometimes viral or bacterial. The neurocellular dimension of these diseases is rarely mentioned, whether in exchanges between medical specialists or explanations destined for the public at large (see appendix 3). Nevertheless, imbalances in (sometimes even exhaustion of) the nervous system and the immune system are always implicated in the appearance and evolution of pathological states, even if the proportions vary from one disease to the next and from one patient to the next.

In reality, it all depends on the way in which we consider, observe, and classify the symptoms of these diseases. The more we move away from the infinitely small to consider systems more and more vast and complex (from the molecular to the tissue level, then to the nervous system, the neuroimmune system, or the neuroimmunohormonal system), the more difficult it becomes to describe the problems linked to these diseases in a purely physiological way without introducing some neuroemotional element.

THE ESSENTIAL ROLE
OF EMOTIONS

Our emotions (all our emotions, from the most violent to the most insignificant) are the center of our mental life. They are closely connected to our nervous system, which itself constantly interacts with our other organic systems and equilibrium. But what is this endless waltz of our neurotransmitters, this psychobiological bridge that connects the virtual world of emotions and thought to the real, material, biological world? The following, if not an example, is at the very least an analogy that seems to clarify this point. When we try to explain motor functions in a purely physiological way (by means of all the organs, muscles, tissues, and body substances that let us move through space), we do so with little difficulty. The cerebral areas responsible for our movements are clearly pinpointed and localized. They react to stimulation in a predictable and repetitive way. Our bodies use zones of neuroreceivers and neurotransmitters, known as synapses (the structures that allow neurons to pass an electrical or chemical signal), connected to movement, but also to seeing, smelling, hearing, and language. When stimulated electrically, they produce certain gestures, reflexes, secretions, and sensations that are codified, predictable, observable, and, therefore, real.

On the other hand, no one has ever succeeded in isolating a "zone of thought" in the brain. Numerous cerebral centers and nuclei allow for the expression of these thoughts (the language zone, the motor functions zone), but thought itself seems to "spread out" through the electrical activity of the entire brain. It's as if the complexity and scope of the processes at work have made any localization impossible—or just "virtually imaginable."

Researchers have likewise never succeeded in locating a "zone of memory" in the brain. Again, there exist areas and relay centers that express our memories and retransmit them, but it is impossible to locate memory itself. In scientific literature numerous researchers describe memory as being a holographic function* of the brain, engaging immense neuronal populations that are individually involved in memory and emotion imagery, leading to memory. So if you have to remember the address of your grandmother's house, where you spent your vacations as a child, your molecular memory will re-create a dozen mental images and offer them as suggestions (like actual photos in a catalog). But in order to select the best image (the right one, that is), you let emotions directly connected to the memory of your grandmother's house intervene, without knowing it. The recollection, the sorting, and the memory choice are always associated with an emotion that you have experienced and that is associated with the memory that you're attempting to recall, to dig up from the stock (the catalog) that constitutes your memory. The emotion homes in on the right photo, or the right image, in your memory. Or, in this case, the right address.

Memory constitutes a sort of "emotional thought." It carries out the incredible transition between neuronal, molecular, and cellular (biochemical and quite real) levels on the one hand, and the emotional or purely virtual on the other. Memory would be impossible without a close, direct relationship to emotion. It is this bridge between emotions and biology that serves as the basis for the vast therapeutic lever of psychoneuroimmunology.

DELTA MEDICINE AND EMOTIONS

Human emotional manifestations are quite varied because they build on a neurophysiological substratum that is constructed from the moment of

---

*The holographic image of an object (or hologram) is composed of thousands of minuscule units that each contain all the information concerning the object. Conversely, a photographic image is composed of thousands of units (points or pixels) more or less dense, each point nothing but an isolated unit, without significance outside the points that surround it. If you rip a photo into little pieces, you will obtain nothing but incomprehensible fragments. If you break a hologram, you will obtain a multitude of fragments, each carrying the entire image. But it seems that there's even more to it with memory: each neuron can develop a unique role, becoming, under certain conditions, a holographic unit of memory.

birth and is enriched by experience over the course of your life. In order to live, a body must receive air and food by eating and breathing. It must also receive multiple sources of external stimulation so that it develops nervous, hormonal, and immune systems. But much of this information is, of necessity, embedded in emotional phenomena. In return, the emotions created have an impact on all the organs of the body through the nervous system. By voluntarily modifying our way of thinking (positive thinking, creative thinking, guided mental imagery), by working on soothing our emotions, and by rebalancing our overall psychoemotional functioning, we can strengthen our nervous, hormonal, and immune equilibrium. The human being is a whole, whose different elements are separately observable but functionally indistinguishable from one another. Psychoemotional functioning has an impact on the body's equilibrium, and the organic functioning has an impact on the psychoemotional equilibrium.* This is why Delta Medicine insists on the importance of integrating this indispensable neuroemotional dimension; its effectiveness alone equals that of the other Delta techniques combined. But in my experience patients often focus on nutrition, breathing, and the detox program (which, in some ways, recalls the "magic potions" of herbalists), and the mind-body approach and management of emotions are deliberately neglected. If you want this book to fulfill its promise, be sure to devote equal time, motivation, and regular practice to all the Delta techniques, including Delta Relaxation (Tool #4) and Delta Psychology (Tool #5). They are fundamental and indispensable.

WORDS CAN WEIGH YOU DOWN

Working on emotions is very important, particularly when you hear the frightening words, *You have cancer, You have multiple sclerosis,* or *You*

---

*Delta Medicine proposes using positive, observable connections between the body and the mind, even if they are difficult to explain, in order to promote everything that reinforces the mind-body equilibrium. Or put more simply: Do what's good for the body, mind, and spirit!

have an autoimmune disease. The relationship patients maintain with their illness builds on these first words. Nobody can dispute the power of words at that moment to shape the thoughts and emotions associated with them.

The doctor-patient relationship can be marked from the beginning by the words attached to the disease and the emotional tone as the doctor pronounces them. The announcement of cancer still remains especially dramatic, because in spite of any therapeutic advances, the term itself is associated with the idea of an unfavorable, or even fatal, prognosis. The shock produced by the announcement of the diagnosis is progressively modulated by certain objective elements: the degree of seriousness, the stage, how aggressive the cancer is, and the prognosis the doctor can reasonably give. The shock is equally influenced by subjective factors. The way the doctor or medical team opens that first dialogue profoundly influences the way the patient will navigate the therapeutic voyage that awaits, the severity of the treatments, side effects, fatigue, and the like. But those who work in the medical profession don't have enough time to devote to this announcement, and they don't have the time to invest the emotional energy necessary to form a relationship with the patient, which may figure prominently in the quality and effectiveness of the overall therapy. They cannot mitigate the immediate or long-term consequences of this emotional deficit. These medical professionals concentrate on their competencies and on the expectations of them by the patient community. And this is already an enormous responsibility, one that numerous specialists have described as "superhuman."

One thing seems certain: the medical truth must be told. (An aside: In very rare cases, the weakened psychological state of the patient doesn't allow for this kind of truth-telling. However, this is the exception, not the rule.) Delta Medicine cannot fulfill its role if patients aren't holding all the cards. They must know what is happening inside the body, what the risks are, and what they will have to confront and go through.*

---

*Interestingly, this medical truth may spark in patients certain beneficial reactions, including a sense of combativeness.

But this doesn't mean that we can dump this hard reality on a person without softening the blow, without drawing on the psychological relationship established between doctor and patient.* The impact will be different depending on the words used, the tone employed, the way things are presented, the moment chosen. Being a therapist, a simple human being who is kind and willing to listen, doesn't come without training. Mind-body medical techniques work, but they are too often neglected in medical university coursework. Working on ourself, working on our emotional and relationship abilities, is so much more difficult than acquiring the knowledge that allows access to the enviable status of "the one who knows."

Nevertheless, this is something to be aware of: certain words carry with them the hope of life, while others connote such negativity that they leave the patient shaken and deeply depressed. Beyond these words and of equal importance is the emotional tone of the doctor. The vocabulary tied to serious illnesses often sets off profound emotions because these words are closely associated with the idea of duration (treatments are long and life suddenly seems short), hardship (numerous and sometimes brutal side effects), and social dislocation (the patient has to make drastic life changes). The vocabulary of illness often carries a sense of drama and fatalism. This is the case with cancer, with its tenacious image as an incurable, painful disease, which, as I will reiterate many times in this book, is false. This common image endures, in spite of the progress that has allowed us to lengthen the average life of patients and considerably increase the number of remissions, and even complete recoveries, for certain types of cancer.

UNDERSTAND, THEN LIGHTEN THE LOAD

That first emotional impact, whose negative effect on the course of the illness is undeniable, can be diminished with the explanations that

---

*I hope that my colleagues will forgive me for broaching the essential and delicate subject of the doctor-patient relationship. I do so in a spirit of openness and in all respect.

Delta Medicine provides about the genesis and evolution of disease.* Once patients understand that they have a standard genetic code, that they were born in good health, and that by using Delta techniques they can regain their good health, they are better able to place in perspective the label "sick" that has suddenly been affixed to them. Patients can then return to a less frightening reality. They discover that their cells (which need to eat, breathe, and receive sustenance from the hormonal and immune systems every day) have suffered from such an accumulation of imbalances that the sick side of their life balance has ended up heavier than the healthy side. Symptoms have appeared, allowing the medical profession to name the illness, to affix that famous label: the diagnosis. It is a simple label, and certainly necessary, but it has nothing to do with inevitability.

This awareness, this new understanding, diminishes feelings of injustice. The bitter sentiment, "Why me?" is often a source of useless, destructive anger. If you can simply answer the question like this— "Because imbalances have accumulated in my life scale"—it short-circuits deleterious emotions. This multifactorial illness has built itself, little by little, inside your body, without your realizing the multitude of small imbalances that were accumulating. So you shouldn't feel responsible for or guilty about this, even if you were the involuntary agent of its construction. We have said it before: it isn't your fault if an illness has developed within you. Your cells, tissues, and organs have simply become victims of pollution, imbalances, and repeated behavioral missteps. That doesn't imply that you are guilty of actions that brought on the illness. Rather, it implies that you are a victim, but a victim who

---

*Any other detailed explanations that are kind, reasonably lucid, and optimistic can be equally useful when offered by a doctor who sets aside the time to do so. In general, doctors who are abrupt or curt have not succeeded in taming their own fears in the face of illness. Try to be forgiving of their insensitivity. Nevertheless, you don't have to be subjected to these doctors. They are themselves "blocked" at the level of this behavior, using their abruptness as a defense mechanism. Try to broaden the dialogue by politely explaining what is hurting or shocking you, as well as your hopes and expectations. Such an attitude can only help both of you as you take this journey together.

is able to react from the moment you understand the origin of these imbalances and mistakes. And as a victim who understands and acts, you can become the agent of your own recovery, just as you are, in part, the agent of your illness.

You thus become a conscious agent of your better welfare, although you were previously not conscious of your imbalances. And this difference has a considerable impact, because it counters the numerous fears associated with the disease.

CANCER: PRIVILEGED TERRITORY OF FEAR

By pushing back the boundaries of the unknown, the unexplainable, and the unjust, Delta Medicine helps drive away fear.

According to theories of modern psychology, fear and anxiety are not identical. Fear is linked to an objective cause outside of ourself, while anxiety is fueled by an interior fear, an idea or a repressed memory that acts in hidden ways. With serious illness, and especially with cancer, these two emotions—fear and anxiety—join together, merge, and feed on each other. The objective, external cause (I am sick and in danger of dying, or at least my life is in danger) serves as a catalyst to the interior, imprecise, secret anxiety (all the fears and repressed emotions are then reactivated).

This anxiety, which we all bear to some extent, depending on our degree of neurosis, takes root in our identity as mortals. Our unconscious, which lives as if we were an immortal entity, doesn't want to accept what constitutes, paradoxically, our only certitude as living beings: we are going to die one day. The fear of death is thus always at the root of anxiety. Confronted with a serious disease, especially cancer, which is so tightly intertwined in our collective unconscious with the idea of death, we let this deep, ancestral anxiety rise to the surface, propelled by an assortment of objective elements (diagnosis, treatment, reaction from the medical profession). Again, understanding the workings of the illness and being able to act consciously defuse this fear and the anxieties linked to it. This allows for a reversal of the negative current prompted by the announcement of the illness and makes way for the reconstruction of emotional stability.

I conclude this essential passage with a thought from author Barry Long (*Only Fear Dies*) that is full of strength, maturity, and courage: "In dying daily to my unhappiness, dying for life, I finally realize the incredible truth: There is no death. All that dies is my fear of dying. Only fear dies. And the death of fear is liberation."

I often quote this to my patients. They derive strength from it, the pure energy of this incredible realization. Cancer and all degenerative diseases return us to the "death idea" that is socially imprinted in our unconscious. Accept it, but only so that your fear will die. You want to live—to learn again to live, perhaps—but to live.

REPLACE THE SCARY WORDS

To ease my patients' unavoidable anxiety produced by disease, I resolved back when I began my medical practice to take the time necessary to explain the reality of the facts of each diagnosis. But I also applied a modified vocabulary, particularly when talking about cancer and serious diseases with dire-sounding medical names.

When a doctor observes in a patient an increased erythrocyte sedimentation rate (an essential test for inflammation) associated with a suspicious mass somewhere in the body, the doctor diagnoses the illness (after further analysis) using the two most widespread terms: *tumor* and *cancer*. In the same way, when that doctor observes a modification in the full blood count, with a lower number of red blood cells associated with an abnormal increase in white blood cells, he will talk about *leukemia* (after additional tests). These words scare people because of their strong emotional charge; they are easily associated with drama, helplessness, and suffering. So I decided once and for all to avoid repeating these terms, the bearers of anxiety and disastrous prognoses, without distorting reality or minimizing what lies ahead.

Once the diagnosis is made and explained, I prefer to speak of *cellular problems* during follow-up consultations.

Delta Medicine is not intended for one particular disease with a scary name: it concerns a group of vital systems, and it strives to revitalize and support their functioning. So we can, without lying or sugarcoating the facts, categorize all cancers, as well as degenerative and autoimmune diseases, as *cellular problems*. The goal isn't to hide the truth from the patient, nor to mask it; quite the contrary. Each patient I treat clearly knows the disease that affects him as well as its workings. But this relabeling makes it possible to avoid the scary words and lessen the anxiety associated with them.* It helps the patient modify his relationship to the illness.

Not only is the term *cellular problem* considerably less dire-sounding than the term *cancer* (or *serious disease X* or *Y*), it is also less weighted with images of helplessness, suffering, and drama. It holds within it a grain of hope and a possible solution. A *cellular problem* relates, as its name indicates, to a dysfunction in the process of cellular construction. So a response exists, a "cellular solution": the deconstruction of that which slowly built itself up within the hidden recesses of the body. A problem that has a solution makes the patient feel much more in control and optimistic about the future, on both the conscious and unconscious levels.

Once the medical diagnosis is clearly made, changing the vocabulary has another positive effect on patients: it helps them feel that they are the agents of their illness, just as they will later be the agents of their health. This is an essential realization, and a considerable aid over the course of the treatment and on the path to recovery: our illness belongs to us. It's detestable, it makes its negative imprint on us, we'd like to vomit it out, to yank it from our body. But it belongs to us. In realizing

---

*Perhaps you have had a similar experience: if you go to work with a mild fever, all it takes is four or five people telling you, "You look terrible today!" and the day will be that much more difficult to get through. Those who claim that words have no influence on emotions and daily well-being are either kind liars or cruel tricksters!

this, patients can stop considering their sick organs as enemies within or traitors to be beaten and view them rather as weakened entities they will strive to support. This is another essential step on the path to awakening our healing forces.

Take, for example, breast cancer. The idea of the "enemy organ" is so strong that some women are relieved to undergo a mastectomy, even when it involves a complete amputation of the breast. They feel as if they have rid themselves of an undesirable host, something "bad." It's as if they have confused the target organ with the affliction itself. Such an attitude compounds the difficulties generated by illness. This sense of liberation prompts patients to be content with the surgery. They obediently follow the chemotherapy, hormone therapy, or radiation therapy regimens with resignation. They make no modifications in how they go about their daily lives and do nothing to change the (accessible, everyday) imbalances that have contributed to the internal construction of the illness, thus depriving themselves of an essential tool for healing. On a psychoemotional level, the idea of considering part of ourself the enemy or a traitor slows the therapeutic reconciliation between body, thoughts, and emotions. It is this reconciliation that forms the core of Delta Medicine techniques.

One last remark: This bad (and common) reflex to project negative feelings onto one part of our body can be even more damaging in the case of autoimmune diseases, which the medical profession describes as follows: "One part of your body rebels against itself and progressively destroys your entire organism." What a terrible association. The therapeutic response of Tool #4 (Delta Relaxation) would be a very valuable aid in this case.

PUT AN END TO ADDICTIVE BEHAVIORS

A few words about the individual's role in the construction of disease: The imbalances and bad habits that accumulate on the sick side of our life balance often occur outside our conscious awareness. As I emphasized earlier, nobody is guilty of not knowing how to breathe properly or of consuming a diet too heavy in industrial pollutants. Nevertheless, certain behaviors are known and largely denounced for their negative impact on the body: smoking, excessive consumption of alcohol, overeating, unmanaged stress, and emotions pushed to the extreme. The damaging effects of these behaviors are covered in the media on a regular basis, to the point that no one can ignore them. And yet some people don't stop these behaviors, thus playing an active and conscious part in the eventual construction of disease in their bodies.

Of course, we are no longer talking about involuntary behaviors here. Each of us must take responsibility for our addictive behaviors. Doctors and the media must continue to inform us, and do so better and better. But we must never point our finger at those who don't resist the temptation of an addiction, nor implicate only their willpower, or lack thereof, in this story. Addictive behaviors (drinking, smoking, anorexia, bulimia) often escape the force of individual willpower, because they are anchored deep inside the mind. The mechanisms of addiction and dependency render addicts prisoner to the point that it is difficult, or even impossible, for them to break free of these addictions by force of willpower alone. We'd all like to have enough willpower to face life's trials and travails with grace and finesse. Through the simple, progressive work on thoughts and emotions (Tools #4, Delta Relaxation, and #5, Delta Psychology), Delta Medicine can help you take those first steps toward ending dependency. It may not be enough to permanently break the vicious cycle of addiction, but it's an impetus to help you embark on that journey to liberation and healing.

IT'S ALWAYS POSSIBLE TO ACT

When diverse imbalances converge in a cluster to disrupt our profound equilibrium, they put our health in jeopardy. Take, for example, nutritional imbalances. Chemical additives and industrial pollutants hidden in some foods are difficult to avoid without returning to a diet close to that of our great-grandparents, which would cause complete social isolation—no restaurant meals of any kind, never a meal outside the house, never a quick meal. But one single source of imbalance (in this case, nutritional contaminants) doesn't suffice in the construction of an illness; there must be several. And it's always possible to counteract certain elements of this disease-causing cluster. This is one of the essential points of Delta Medicine.

Breathing better, for example, is something everyone can do; so is improving our management of stress and emotions by way of small adjustments and simple rituals. Whatever the organization or rhythm of our lives, whatever the degree of pollution in our environment, whatever the events or changes we experience, it's always possible to voluntarily contribute to the prevention of disorders, to work to reverse the movement that has made the life balance tip to the side of illness.

A PROGRESSIVE PROGRAM

Serious diseases—cancer, in particular—lead patients into infernal, negative circles, lessening their chances of healing. The emotional shock set off by the announcement of the disease causes underlying psychoemotional disorders to resonate. The loss of appetite brought on by some treatments adds to the imbalances and nutritional bad habits that contributed to the genesis of the disorder. These are only a few of the most common examples.

Delta Medicine breaks this morbid spiral by focusing our attention on healthier and more appropriate behaviors. But that means that our investment in these healing practices must follow a regular progression. If we slam down on the accelerator of a car before warming up the motor, there is a good chance that we will damage the engine. It's the same for our body. Taking gradual, progressive steps is all the more important because the body is an infinitely more complex and subtle "machine" than a car.

The progression in this book follows two overarching phases:

- During the first, it rebalances and reprograms the metabolism.
- Then, during the second, we can call on healing forces without the risk of asking too much of the body, which is now more balanced but still convalescent.

The harmonization, the reprogramming of the body's functions, must always precede their support, and then their stimulation.

Each of the following "Tools" chapters is dedicated to one of the five basic techniques of Delta Medicine. You will find specific advice on the practice itself and on the progressive phases that you will need to follow to integrate that tool in your healing regimen. Resist the temptation to accelerate the tempo and rush through them. Remain concerned but patient, in the true sense of the word. The results will be deeper and longer-lasting. Be confident, motivated, and consistent in your practice.

Some people favor one technique and skip the others. However, if you fail to give each of the techniques equal weight, you will limit the effectiveness of Delta Medicine.

So be motivated and aware of the three forces, the three grounds of healing that make up your being: body, mind, and spirit. You now know that tools for health dedicated to all three of these grounds do exist.

Practice each technique to some extent every day, each with the same resolve. This is Delta Medicine.

You are about to begin a program to deconstruct your illness and reconstruct yourself.

Key Points

→ The five techniques of Delta Medicine presented in this book, taken individually, have been studied in hospitals and applied in numerous countries (Canada, United States, Belgium, Germany, Japan).

→ None of these techniques alone can cure cancer or an autoimmune or degenerative disease. It is in conjunction with contemporary medical treatments that they realize their effectiveness.

→ Our emotions play an essential role in our biological equilibrium and in the maintenance of our health. Working on emotions is particularly important because the announcement of a serious illness often generates a flood of negative, destructive emotions that individuals must learn to regulate.

→ The announcement of a serious disease often sets off a flood of feelings of injustice that are difficult to combat. Understanding the actions, behaviors, and feelings that implicate us in the construction of the illness helps us reverse the progress of illness and return to good health.

→ Fear is also omnipresent when people learn that they have a serious illness. To avoid exacerbating this fear, as soon as the diagnosis is made and explained I advise both doctors and patients to systematically refrain from using the term *cancer,* instead referring to the illness as a *cellular problem.* Why? Because a problem often has a *solution.* And this gives patients—both consciously and unconsciously—hope and motivation.

→ Delta Medicine helps patients make peace with the sick organ, instead of outright rejecting it. In reality, this weak link signals all our imbalances. It deserves to be supported and even thanked: this is one of the axes of Delta Relaxation.

→ Whatever our state of health, it's always possible to act, get involved, participate, and be the agent of healing by tipping the scale to the healthy side of our life balance.

→ Delta Medicine's advice about the program's techniques and practices follows a progressive order.

→ In all cases, it's important to first rebalance the metabolism in order to stimulate our healing energies; that is, program ourself to heal.

→ Respect this program and, above all, devote the same amount of time and attention to each of the five tools of Delta Medicine. This is the key to their coordinated effectiveness, and the key to your healing process.

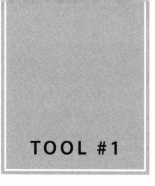

TOOL #1

DELTA BREATHING

Most of us have never received instruction about breathing and how to take advantage of it as a harmonizer of mind and body. . . . Breathing may be the master function of our body, affecting all others.

DR. ANDREW WEIL, *SPONTANEOUS HEALING*

"Slow your breath . . . more . . . more . . . There, look at the curve of your cardiac rhythm!" Guided by Paul Lehrer, the scientist conducting the experiment, the patient then sees the curve on the screen become smooth, its oscillation grow, and its rhythm stabilize. "Maintain this respiratory rhythm so that the sinusoid [the curve shaped like an ocean swell that translates the heartbeat onto a video screen] remains regular," the researcher continues. The session lasts twenty minutes.

"After ten weeks of these twice-weekly sessions," he explains, "the volunteers reduce the doses of their medication by one-third. And the number of attacks they experience is half that compared to a test group of twenty-three asthma patients not doing the exercises."

This experiment, reported in a major scientific magazine,* is one

---

*Extract of an article titled "Concentration on Biorhythms Cures Asthma," published in *Science et Vie (Science and Life),* no. 1046 (November 2004).

of many examples of the therapeutic power of standardized breathing exercises.

I have chosen to introduce the breathing technique first, as Delta Tool #1, because it immediately offers several advantages. First, you can start practicing it right away. You don't need to make big changes in your life: you're not changing what you put in your cart at the supermarket, nor are you changing the way you typically manage stress and bad news. All it takes is five short minutes to start doing the first breathing exercise.

Second advantage: The Delta Breathing technique acts rapidly on a neurovascular level, and its benefits are noted immediately in terms of your well-being. It also eases the brutal emotional shock related to the announcement of a disease.

A BRIDGE BETWEEN BODY AND MIND

Humans can survive several weeks without eating and several days without drinking, but we cannot spend more than several minutes without breathing (except for those who are trained at it). Of all the forms of nourishment indispensable to us, air is the most important and the most abundant. Each day we absorb about 2 pounds of solid food, 4 pounds of liquids (beverages and foods combined), and nearly 18 pounds of air! Our breath is the thin but powerful thread that connects us to life, from the first second of our existence until the moment we "draw our last breath." Our life on this planet begins when we take our first inhalation and stretch our little lungs to receive this gaseous food, thus allowing our cells to transform the "nutritional fuel" of our daily food into energy and organic structure. Adenosine triphosphate (ATP) is our body's fundamental unit of energy. It is what gives our cells the strength to form before giving us the strength to move. Without breathing and its precious contribution of oxygen, it would be impossible for us to produce ATP.

One undeniable sign of the vital importance of breath is the way breathing figures in our daily vocabulary and many current expressions. For example, we talk about *a second wind* to express a renewal of energy after a moment of fatigue that leaves us *out of breath*. Those prone to exaggerate are *full of hot air,* but just like the rest of us, they can *gasp* with emotion. They'd better not *hold their breath,* though, if they're expecting a *breathtaking* scene of beauty.

We breathe between twelve and eighteen times a minute throughout our life. This represents 600 to 700 million inhalations and exhalations over the course of an average life span (more than a billion for those who live to one hundred). We breathe day and night, at rest and on the move, whether we're sick or well (but not with the same frequency, nor the same amplitude). Most of the time we do so without thinking about it: our chest rises, our diaphragm contracts, the volume of our thoracic cage increases and air penetrates our lungs. Then, inside our body, gaseous exchanges allow the blood to load up with oxygen and get rid of carbon dioxide. Finally, the thoracic cage falls, our diaphragm expands, and the carbon dioxide–laden air is expelled from the body.

We don't need to pay attention to our breath for it to give rhythm to our existence. But breathing possesses a particularity that makes it unique: all we need to do is focus our attention on our breath to control it, to take over the automatic piloting of our brain. We can slow or accelerate the rhythm of our breathing and increase or reduce its amplitude at will and without much effort. It is our only vital function to enjoy this privilege. Our heart beats without our thinking about it, but our will seems to have no effect on its rhythm.* On the other hand, our movements are the fruit of our conscious thinking. We cannot move without deciding to: our motor muscles do not contract in the absence of intentional orders.

So breathing bridges the divide between the conscious world and the depths of the unconscious. We have all experienced the connection

---

*Interestingly, we'll see later on that the reality is actually much more complex: by controlling our breathing and our thoughts, we can impact our cardiac rhythm.

between breathing and cardiac rhythm in an intuitive way. Just by voluntarily calming the breath (especially on the exhale), the beating of the heart will immediately calm, too. At the same time, a beneficial warmth, a sense of well-being, even peace, progressively sweeps over the body and mind. Under certain conditions, breathing can become a link between body, thoughts, and emotions. Ever since the time of Hippocrates, medical practitioners from all eras and in all countries have understood and widely exploited this in therapy. We will return to this point later.

When better controlled, our breath can enhance our metabolic and cardiovascular functions as well as our psychoemotional equilibrium. This is what makes breathing (as a voluntary act) an irreplaceable tool in the maintenance of our health, a tool able to strongly influence the oscillations of the life balance on each side of the Delta Point (see the chapter titled "The Construction and Deconstruction of Illness"). Alas, we tend to forget this and allow breathing to proceed mostly as an unconscious, involuntary action, rather than a conscious action. As long as it doesn't become the source of a pathological imbalance (a respiratory affliction, such as emphysema or asthma), we prefer to direct our attention and energies to other mind-body practices. Most of the time we consider our breathing a reflex, while we could be using it as an essential tool to improve our well-being and maintain our health.

HOW WE BREATHE

Who impulsively worries about breathing the right or wrong way, superficially or deeply, rapidly or slowly? Yet breathing plays an essential role in all our vital functions. Its first goal is to bring the central life element, oxygen, to all our cells. The respiratory function thus figures in all vital exchanges, because it nourishes all the tissues of the body: the brain and nervous system, the sensory organs (eyes, skin, mucous membranes), the digestive organs (stomach, liver, intestines), the endocrine glands (adrenal, ovaries, thyroid), and the bones, muscles, and joints.

We absorb the air that surrounds us in its totality, but we use just one component of this vital gaseous mixture—oxygen. Air is mainly composed of nitrogen (78 percent), mixed with oxygen (21 percent) and traces of rare gases (helium, krypton, neon). Nitrogen is a neutral gas that "softens" the action of oxygen. Thankfully, because oxygen is very reactive. If we breathed pure oxygen, it would react so violently with our living cells that Earth's surface would be rapidly deprived of life (or of ours, at least). By breathing, we draw the optimum amount of oxygen from the air, which is then used as fuel inside each cell in a small energy station called the mitochondria.

Thanks to this oxygen, the mitochondria transform the other principal fuel that supplies nourishment—glucose—into ATP (adenosine triphosphate). ATP is our true life unit. We often hear that oxygen is life. But, in reality, ATP is life. It's our primary source of energy: without this specific energy molecule, life would not be possible, movements could not be made, and, above all, human structure could not take shape.

On a strictly anatomical level, we breathe thanks to a structure made of bones, muscles, ligaments, tendons, and various types of mucus—the thoracic cage (see figure on page 52). By modifying its volume, the thoracic cage allows the lungs to expand and contract. (Contrary to popular misconceptions, the lungs do not breathe. It is the thoracic cage and the powerful diaphragmatic muscle that make them breathe.) The lungs sit inside this cage, formed of ribs that fit into the vertebral column in the back. On the upper part of the torso, the ribs form arches that join at the center of the chest and come together at the sternum. On the lower part, the ribs are shorter. The last two are said to be "floating" because they aren't attached to any structure on the front side of the body. The lungs are "stuck" to the thoracic cage by a special tissue called the pleura. When the pleura becomes infected and inflamed, this causes the infamous disease known as pleurisy. The ribs are separated by intercostal muscles; releasing and contracting causes them to spread apart or come together, modifying the volume of our thorax.

An astonishing flat, horizontal muscle closes the thoracic cage at its lowest point; this is the diaphragm. It's attached to the lower ribs, the vertebrae, and the sternum, forming a sort of floor, and it separates the thorax from the abdominal cavity below it, where the principal organs of the digestive system, among other organs, are housed.

Safe inside this cozy nest, the lungs are protected from potential blows. When we inhale, the ribs spread apart and the diaphragm expands. This additional space forces the lungs to fill with air. When

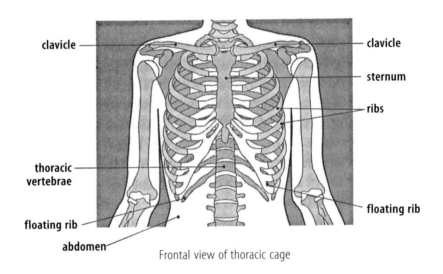

Frontal view of thoracic cage

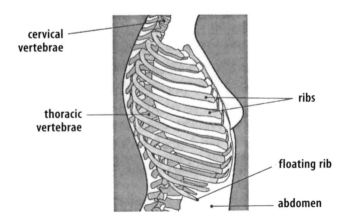

Profile view of thoracic cage

we exhale, the ribs compress and the diaphragm contracts. The volume of the thoracic cage decreases and the lungs empty like a sponge squeezed between your fingers to wring out water.

WHY DO WE BREATHE?

Let's go inside the lungs. We have two of them, of different sizes. The left lung is a bit less roomy than the right one because it must make room for the heart, so we have two lobes in the left lung as opposed to three in the right lung.

The respiratory apparatus resembles an upside-down tree whose branches reach toward the ground. The trachea, a tube through which air travels from the nose and mouth, forms the trunk of this tree. The trachea then divides into two bronchi, which divide into thinner and thinner tubes, the bronchioles. On the thinnest bronchioles hang the little sacks that form the pulmonary tissue—the alveoli. Each of us possesses about 300 million of them. Laid out on the ground, end to end, they would cover the surface of a tennis court! A truly giant surface, but indispensable to executing the hundreds of millions of cellular exchanges necessary with each breath.

When you inhale, air enters through your nose or mouth (preferably your nose, because it filters, humidifies, and warms the air) and then travels through the trachea, the bronchi, and the bronchioles to get to the alveoli, which inflate. It is inside the minuscule pulmonary alveoli that the first vital gaseous exchanges are made. The alveoli's extremely fine walls are surrounded by a network of microscopic vessels, called capillaries. The contaminated blood, loaded with cellular waste, is led to these capillaries by the pulmonary artery.* The carbon dioxide contained in the contaminated blood passes through the walls

---

*This artery is the only vessel in the body called an "artery" although it carries blood rich in carbon dioxide. The term *artery* is normally reserved for vessels that transport blood rich in oxygen; the others, with carbon dioxide, are called "veins."

and into the pulmonary alveoli. At the same time, the oxygen travels in the opposite direction, from the alveoli into the bloodstream. Cleaned of its gaseous waste and charged with the precious oxygen that fastens to the hemoglobin molecules, the blood leaves for the pulmonary veins[*] and proceeds to the heart, which contracts to propel the blood into the entire circulatory system.

This operation keeps occurring, between twelve and eighteen times a minute for the breathing and between sixty and seventy-five times a minute for the beating of the heart, during our entire life. These cycles ensure the number-one function of breathing: to transport to the cells the indispensable oxygen needed for cellular metabolism and to rid the body of the carbon dioxide produced by that cellular metabolism. At the same time, the blood releases other wastes, notably part of its surplus of acidity, because in order to function well our internal environment must remain moderately acidic.

Even a slight increase in this internal acidity brings with it numerous long-term health problems:[†] the disturbed circulatory system hinders the nourishment of the cells as well as the regular elimination of metabolic waste. In the short term, acidity attacks the tissues, which promotes latent microinflammatory states favorable to cellular problems (as well as degenerative troubles).[‡]

The internal acidity rate is regulated by complex mechanisms. The twentieth century saw tissue hyperacidity take hold, promoted by progressive imbalances in our diet in addition to the inhuman rhythms of modern life and the omnipresent pressures of daily stress. In combination with a slight nutritional adjustment (see the chapter on Tool #2,

---

[*]These "veins" are the only ones in the body to receive blood rich in oxygen; the name *veins* is ordinarily reserved for vessels through which blood with carbon dioxide circulates. This is the "pulmonary exception."

[†]I'm not talking here about the illness called metabolic acidosis, but rather a chronic tissue acidity that paves the way for numerous degenerative diseases.

[‡]For more on this subject, see the excellent work by Dr. Christopher Vasey, *The Acid–Alkaline Diet for Optimum Health* (Rochester, Vt.: Healing Arts Press, 2006).

Delta Nutrition) and regular detoxification of the body (see the chapter on Tool #3, Delta Detoxification), the Delta Breathing exercises can contribute to effectively regulating the degree of internal acidity by modifying the rhythm and intensity of gaseous exchanges.

Respiratory control also curbs the production of free radicals, those hyperactive particles that promote premature aging and numerous cellular disorders. By slowing respiratory rhythm, we diminish the contribution of oxygen to the system. Even though this gas is indispensable to life, it is equally responsible for deleterious cellular hyperoxidation phenomena. The excess of oxygen ions is as harmful as their lack. The controlled slowing of the breath brings with it a limited but useful slowdown in the production of free radicals and promotes a gentle correction of mitochondrial functions. While this may curb the acceleration of the process of cellular aging, it also supports our immune functions (because mitochondrial calming is associated with the good condition of our cellular defenses). These many beneficial effects promote the stabilization of our metabolism and the regression, or the deconstruction, of cellular problems.

CALM THE HEART, STRESS, TENSIONS, AND EMOTIONS

Key action: Controlled breathing has an almost immediate impact on cardiac rhythm. Remember: I explained earlier that we cannot, by sheer force of our will, accelerate or slow our cardiac rhythm. But we can do so indirectly by controlling our breath.

The simple act of breathing (and especially exhaling) more slowly, deeply, and calmly slows the heartbeat within a few seconds. Anyone can confirm this by placing the tips of the index and middle fingers of the right hand on the inside of the left wrist, just below the thumb (see figure on page 56), to feel the change in the heart's rhythm. This slowing can also induce a slight lowering of arterial pressure. So the entire cardiovascular system benefits from this cardiac reprieve.

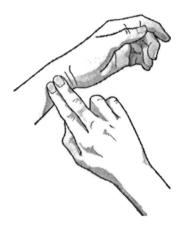

The correct position of the fingers on the wrist to feel the pulse

This respiratory control and the cardiac calming that ensues together contribute to calming both muscular and nervous tensions. When we slow our respiratory rhythm by halving the number of breaths per minute (for example, from fourteen to seven), we quickly notice that mental functioning calms, ideas slow their frenetic racing, and stress loosens its grip. Our emotions then follow this overall positive direction.

I am sure you have already noticed the close relationship between the breath and emotions. Fear and joy both accelerate the breath, making it short and shallow, and can sometimes even suspend it for several seconds; hence the expression *It took my breath away.* Negative emotional changes always play a role in the construction of illness,* a role further amplified by the violent emotional shock that comes with the announcement of a serious disease. Practicing controlled breathing allows you to gently diminish these negative emotional impacts, without pressure or additional stress. We will see later how valuable this is in supporting and enhancing the techniques of Delta Relaxation (Tool #4) and Delta Psychology (Tool #5).

---

*I insist on this term *construction* because it allows for a better understanding of the effectiveness of the Delta Medicine techniques. Stress, nutrition, and emotions are not the disease, but their imbalances anchor the disease to the point that it becomes chronic. And what we construct we can *deconstruct.*

These respiratory exercises are simple and fast-acting—both big advantages. The results that we obtain through regular practice might almost seem like magic if we weren't familiar with the modes of the biophysiological actions responsible for them.

Working on the breath plays a part in mind-body techniques: by acting on a physiological function (the breath), we obtain a calming effect on a physical level (muscular tensions) and on an organic level (cardiac rhythm), as well as on a neuroemotional level (the impact of stress on emotions). Thanks to the training of a bodily function we can fight excess stress and positively influence our nervous tensions and emotions.

WHERE AND WHEN TO PRACTICE DELTA BREATHING

Breathing techniques exist as much in Eastern rituals as in the Western medical clinic. Countless mind-body methods incorporate work on the breath. During my thirty years of observation, I have encountered dozens of techniques, and from them I have selected a very simple type of breathing, easy to practice at any age and in all circumstances, that exerts the maximum beneficial influence on all the parameters we have discussed.

While priority is given to particular postures for practicing certain kinds of age-old breathing techniques (notably yoga and Zen meditation), you can utilize Delta Breathing in any circumstance, even while standing in the middle of a crowded commuter train or bus, provided that you concentrate (and, of course, hold on so that you don't fall when the bus or subway car lurches suddenly). There is only one situation in which you absolutely must avoid doing this practice: while driving a motor vehicle. Even stuck in a traffic jam, you must remain vigilant so that you can react to what is going on around you. In spite of the stress created by driving, especially in the city, you must avoid indulging in any form of relaxation exercise while you are behind the wheel. On the other hand, as a passenger, nothing stops you from practicing Delta Breathing.

This first Delta technique doesn't demand a lot of time. Five minutes will suffice, but you must practice it regularly, two or three times a day. In order to do this, you must find (or create) calm moments in different day-to-day life situations—your health depends on it. At the office or at home, when it's difficult to find a quiet corner where you won't be disturbed, you can always take refuge in the bathroom. This solution often proves useful in the world of work, where there's a lack of privacy but no lack of stress. You can practice in the rest room quite easily with the lights out and the door locked.

THE BEST POSTURES

Delta Breathing can be practiced standing, sitting, or lying down. With a wide range of choices, you can always find a posture suited to the situation in which you find yourself. Nevertheless, you should observe certain rules in order to breathe in good conditions.

▲ The Seated Position

This is the simplest for a Westerner, the most immediate, and my favorite.

- Choose a seat that you can't sink into; a straight-back chair without arms is better than an armchair.
- Sit down so that your thighs and calves form a right angle at the knees when your feet are planted flat on the ground. Your feet and your knees should be about a foot apart. You can also cross your feet and fold them under the chair; this very comfortable position is called *secretary style.*
- Sit up straight without forcing yourself and relax your shoulders.
- Place your hands on top of your thighs, palms toward the ceiling, very relaxed. Close your eyes.

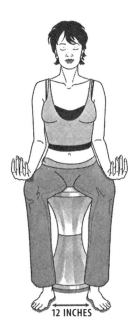

The seated position

12 INCHES

▲ The Coachman Position

I find this position to be just as good as the previous one. Choose the one that works best for you, depending on your body type and how you feel. This position was often used in mind-body medicine in the first half of the twentieth century. It's called the coachman's position because at one time it was regularly adopted by coachmen whose profession required them to remain available over long periods, if not twenty-four hours a day. They didn't have the time to really sleep, so they

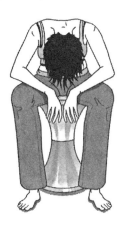

The coachman position

recharged their vital and nervous energies by relaxing (and sometimes, in fact, sleeping) in this position.

- Sit as you did for the previous position and spread your feet a bit farther apart.
- Place your elbows on your thighs, about 5 inches from your knees, and let your hands hang between your legs.
- Then lean forward, curving your back, and let your head hang loose, just above your knees.

This position alone should provide deep relaxation. After several days of trials and adjustments, the first triumph will occur: no part of your body will be tense or tight, and this will occur as soon as you adopt the position.

▲ The Lying-Down Position

This is an excellent position, but less spontaneous. Nevertheless, at the end of the day it promotes sleep better than the seated relaxation. This position remains for many the benchmark of comfortable positions.

- Stretch out on your back on a surface that's neither too firm (you must be comfortable) nor too soft (you must feel supported).
- Let your arms rest loose along the sides of your body and turn your palms to the ceiling.
- Relax your body, especially your neck and shoulders. If you are wearing any tight clothing, unbutton or loosen it to allow more room for your thorax and abdomen to expand, and if you are wearing a belt, loosen it. A man should loosen his tie and unbutton the first few buttons of his shirt if he is wearing a button-down style.

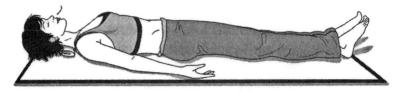

The lying-down position

- Let your head rest naturally, straight, with the back of your head on the ground. You can slide a small, thin pillow under your neck for support, if you wish.
- Close your eyes and relax, with a slight smile (this immediately relaxes the face).

▲ The Standing Position

This is the most difficult position, so do not use it at first. Wait until you have practiced enough with the other postures before trying it.

- Spread your feet apart slightly (about a foot) to brace yourself, your back straight, your shoulders relaxed, your head in line with your vertebral column.
- Tilt your pelvis forward to decrease the curve of your lumbar spine. This will naturally make your knees bend slightly and your buttocks flex.
- Do not close your eyes in order to avoid the risk of falling, but gently lower your eyelids and try to fix your gaze on the ground about 6 feet

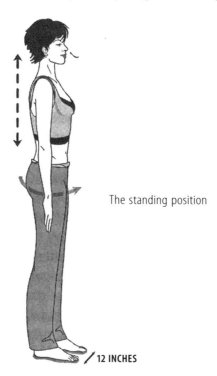

The standing position

12 INCHES

in front of you (this will help remove your consciousness from your external surroundings and focus your attention on the breath).

Again, do not try to adopt this posture during the first few weeks of practice; wait until you are sufficiently used to the breathing technique.

BASIC RULES OF DELTA BREATHING

I'd like to emphasize one fundamental point: the goal of Delta Breathing is not to force your breath, but to give it rhythm, harmony, and ease. It isn't athletic breathing—loud and rapid—nor is it tinged with spirituality, like yoga or Buddhist meditation. This is a physiological practice that will rapidly have an impact on your vital mental and emotional functions. Motivation, regular practice, and respecting the technique are the keys to its effectiveness.

Ideally, you will force yourself (gently and with a smile) to practice three five-minute breathing breaks each day.

- the first one in the morning, when you wake up
- the second one before lunch
- the last one between 8:00 and 9:00 p.m.

You can practice your last breathing exercise of the day just before going to bed, but I recommend that you perform it earlier in the evening, about a half-hour after dinner, so that you can relax and spend the time before you sleep in peace and comfort.

It is very important to always inhale and exhale through the nose (except in one particular case, which I will explain later). The cavities of the nose and the oropharynx (the area of the throat at the back of the mouth) are lined with mucous membranes that warm and humidify the air so that it enters the lungs at the right temperature and degree of moisture. These mucous membranes are also lined with cilia, tiny hairlike organelles that collect some of the impurities contained in the air. It would be a shame to deprive yourself of such an efficient, natural device for cleaning the surrounding air.

Although Delta Breathing is harmonizing and not based on effort, you must still emphasize the exhale a bit by slightly contracting the abdominal muscles and releasing the buttocks (pushing them as if you were going to the bathroom). But be careful: no effort whatsoever must be made on the inhale, which occurs naturally, like the tide that ebbs after touching the shore. The goal of this exercise is, first of all, to divide by two your respiratory rhythm, detoxify your body, and cleanse your system of free radicals. Second, the voluntary lengthening of the exhale calms the cardiovascular system and promotes the circulation of fluids in the brain. When combined with the previous actions, this promotes physical and emotional detoxification.

All these effects will combine to counteract some of the unhealthy phenomena damaging your biological terrain and, in conjunction with conventional treatment, this will help reverse the negative movement of your life balance, prompting it to again lean to the healthy side.

THE FIVE STEPS OF
THE DELTA BREATHING PROGRAM

As I explained earlier, it does no good to fast-forward through the steps. Each phase of the program must be well integrated, both with regard to how you do the exercise and the way in which your metabolism registers and activates the new modes of functioning. Even if you are in pain or anxious to reach a state of well-being, keep in mind that clear-sighted patience during the first seven to ten days of this practice will ensure enduring effectiveness.

The goal is not to reach the last stage as quickly as possible. Rather, it is to give your metabolism the time to rehabilitate, rebalance, and reprogram itself. When you paint the walls of your living room, you must wait for each coat to dry before adding the next one; otherwise, the two coats run into each other and the result is mediocre and less durable. It's the same with your metabolic rehabilitation, whether through Delta Breathing or any of the other Delta techniques presented in this book. Why not start practicing Delta Breathing right now? As soon as you've read the following paragraph, set aside this book and do the first exercise right away.

You will notice a slight soothing effect almost immediately that will help you not only understand but also experience with your own body the important role that breathing plays during every second of your existence. Repeat these breathing exercises seriously over the course of ten days (two weeks for those of you who are more tense): the way you'll feel will remove any urge to abandon this practice!

▲ First Step: Find the Right Rhythm

This first step lasts about ten days, as do all the others. Once you have found a calm place (even the bathroom, if necessary, because you must begin the exercise as soon as possible), settle into the position that works best for you and close your eyes. If you can, practice the coachman posture (page 59) for one minute before starting the exercise in order to completely relax. Then proceed in the following way:

- Start with a deep inhalation (the only one of the entire exercise), followed by a long sigh, mouth open. Let out a vocal sigh—it's not just allowed, it's recommended!
- Then inhale slowly through the nose, this time without forcing it, counting to three (with practice, you will be able to lengthen your inhalation). To avoid counting too quickly, I recommend counting like this: one one thousand, two one thousand, three one thousand. The act of pronouncing the entire number gives a better rhythm to your counting.
- Then exhale very slowly through the nose, slightly forcing your breath and counting up to six (still using the same method of counting: one one thousand, two one thousand, three one thousand).
- Always inhale and exhale through the nose (except for the first breath-sigh).

- Breathe this way for five minutes, trying to focus your attention on the rhythm you give your breath. Concentrate on the air that enters and exits at the base of your nose. Envision it entering and exiting like a "glowing wind."

- Then, if possible, return to the coachman position for one minute before opening your eyes and returning to your normal life.

- Concentrate only on the rhythm of your breathing. Within a few days, once you feel that you are becoming comfortable with the exercise, you can progressively lengthen the time of your inhalation and exhalation, making sure that the exhale is always twice as long as the inhale: if you count up to four (one thousand) while inhaling, you will count up to eight (one thousand) while exhaling, and so on. This lets you amplify the exchange of oxygen in the lungs and increase the flow of toxic discharge.

To time the five minutes necessary for the exercise, I recommend using a soothing song (something classical, or relaxation music), or even the alarm of your cell phone (a good use for a normally stressful object).

▲ Second Step: Promote Abdominal Breathing

Over the course of the following ten days, continue to breathe in this same way, always trying to lengthen your inhale and exhale (without exceeding five for the inhale and ten for the exhale), in order to slow the rhythm of your breathing without demanding effort. But now you are going to slightly change your posture.

- Whether seated, standing, or lying down, place your hand on your stomach, with your thumb at your belly button, and concentrate on this point of contact.

- Try to feel your stomach rising as you inhale and falling as you exhale. This is the key to abdominal breathing. On the inhalation, feel your abdomen inflating first, as the breath then moves up into the thoracic cage.

At this stage you have sufficiently integrated the breathing rhythm to now concentrate on your abdominal breathing. The act of placing your hand on your stomach will help you concentrate more fully on where this originates and on the depth of your breathing.

▲ Third Step: Make the Most of the Pauses

Three weeks have passed. You have now integrated the breathing rhythm and the deep abdominal breathing into your daily routine. During the ten days that follow, you will add an additional element to your exercise regimen.

■ At the end of the inhale, pause briefly, lungs full, before exhaling. This pause must be short, the time it takes to count to three (still counting one one thousand, two one thousand, three one thousand).

■ Then exhale normally, and at the end of the exhale, pause for the same count, lungs empty.

This pause on the exhale must never be painful.

Make this a progressive practice, taking the time necessary to accustom yourself to the new rhythm. This should not demand any effort on your part or provoke the least bit of physical or mental tension. On the contrary, this should relax your body and mind. Note that these pauses must never last longer than three seconds.

▲ Fourth Step:
Reprogram Your Neuromuscular Relaxation

You've now been practicing your three daily exercises for a month: five minutes in the morning, five minutes at lunchtime, and five minutes in the evening. If all is going well, you are used to it (maybe even "hooked" on it), and the practice isn't posing any problems for you. If this isn't the case, continue one or two weeks longer, until you feel perfectly at ease. Then you can move on to the next phase: this integrates simple head and neck movements that will help you release neuromuscular tensions that accumulate with stress.

For this phase you must do the practice standing or sitting. You cannot do these exercises lying down.

■ If you can, start in the coachman position for thirty seconds, then adopt the seated posture, making sure to sit up straight.

■ Without straining—this is very important—slowly turn your head to the right and left (see figure), as if you were saying *no* (the slowness of the movement is also important). Do this three times (this should take you less than thirty seconds), slowly and continually breathing, without straining yourself.

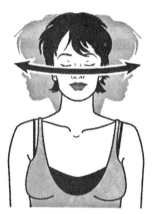

■ Then, still without any strain and very slowly, move your head up and down (see figure), as if you were saying a big *yes* three times (or about thirty seconds), always breathing slowly and without any effort. Pay special attention so that you never strain yourself as you tilt your head backward.

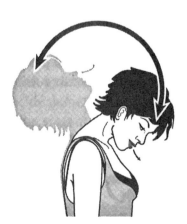

■ Next, still with the same rhythm (slowly and without any strain), tilt your head to the right and to the left, without turning it, as if you wanted to put your ear on your shoulder (see figure). Do this three times (or for about thirty seconds), being careful not to lift your shoulder up to your head (we always do this when standing, as a reflex). The goal is not to make your shoulder and ear touch; that would prove to be difficult unless you are very flexible.

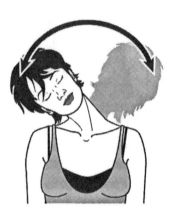

■ Finally, finish this short series of exercises by completely rotating your head, very (very) gently, to the right, then to the left, still breathing very slowly and freely, without straining (see figure). Be sure not to strain when you lean your head toward the back. One single rotation should take about twenty seconds.

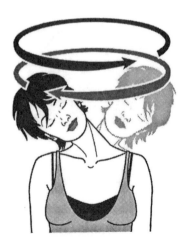

You should never strain or rush when you perform these movements. The movements should never be jerky; rather, they should be done smoothly and with a feeling of ease. And you must add this neuromuscular relaxation preparation to your Delta Breathing only if you feel perfectly at ease with your breathing. The preparation lasts only two minutes, after which you will practice the breathing exercise described above. When you are used to it (after a week or two), you will be able to perform two complete rotations of the head at the end of the preparatory movements, then three (or for about one minute). No more.

These movements are meant to deprogram the neuromuscular tensions that lodge in the zone at the nape of your neck and shoulders, and, often, consequently, in the back. They also gently massage your endocrine glands, located in this part of the body (thymus, thyroid gland), and relax all the nerve paths that go from the brain to the rest of the body. It's the best preparation for Delta Breathing that you could dream of. Try to incorporate it in your program at least twice a day (ideally at the beginning of your Delta Breathing regimen), when you're able to take a little more time and breathe in the seated position.

▲ Fifth (and Last) Step:
A Valuable Variation on the Exhalation

You have been practicing Delta Breathing three times a day for about two months, always inhaling and exhaling through the nose. You will now be able to do what's called the pinched-lips exhalation from time to time.

■ Prepare to breathe as has become your habit and begin your exercise as usual. The only difference lies in the way you exhale.

■ You're going to exhale through the mouth, closing the lips as if you were gently blowing on food that is too hot so as to cool it. Be careful that the stream of air you expel remains fine and does not resemble the puff of air that we use to blow out birthday candles. The inhalation continues as normal, through the nose. This way of exhaling keeps the pulmonary alveoli open under slight pressure in a longer, more dynamic way. It also lets the smallest bronchioles and alveoli dilate. The pulmonary emptying, prompted by this exercise, is deeper and more efficient.

But be aware that this last step must never constitute the entirety of a five-minute breathing session, because this kind of breathing can make your head spin if extended. Be satisfied with exhaling this way four or five times, at the end of an entire breathing exercise.

LATER . . .

Congratulations! These five phases of breathing constitute your first Delta Medicine technique, your first step toward taking control of your overall health and reclaiming your inner harmony. Delta Breathing will start to positively influence your body and program your terrain for deeper detoxification techniques (see the chapter on Delta Detoxication, Tool #3). It will also soothe your neuromuscular system and prepare you for the nervous and emotional balancing exercises in the chapters on Delta Relaxation (Tool #4) and Delta Psychology (Tool #5).

Get in the habit of practicing regularly. The more you do these exercises, the more they will become necessary, in a positive, productive way. As you begin to notice their benefits, the exercises will become indispensable. They also serve as excellent preparation for all the Delta Relaxation and Delta Psychology techniques in the chapters that follow.

Never forget that our breath is our life. Become once again the master of yours, and you will start to take control of your life! Delta Breathing is an essential tool for health. It is the first step on the path to awakening all your healing mechanisms, a first step toward a positive synergy of all your treatments. And as a wise man named Lao-tzu once said, "A journey of a thousand miles starts with one step."

So start now. It's up to you.

Key Points

↦ Delta Breathing is a therapy of the breath. You can rapidly feel its benefits: all it takes is the decision to do it and a few minutes to derive its first positive effects.

↦ The breath is the thread that connects us to life, from our first inhalation when we come into the world until our last breath. According to certain criteria (notably rhythm and amplitude), our breathing can weigh on the healthy side or the sick side of our life balance.

↦ Breathing figures in all our vital functions, all our metabolic exchanges, as well as our psychoemotional balance.

↦ Air constitutes our first form of nourishment. The oxygen it contains allows our cells to transform the glucose from food into energy.

↦ Breathing allows our blood to be replenished with oxygen and dispel carbon dioxide and cellular waste. By controlling amplitude and respiratory rhythm, we can make these exchanges more productive, accelerate the elimination of polluted air that stagnates in the pulmonary tissues, and regulate the acid-alkaline equilibrium in the body (which is responsible, in part, for our health).

↦ We constantly breathe without paying attention to this process. But we can also control our breath if we want to. This makes our respiratory function unique among our autonomic, or involuntary, nervous system functions.

↦ The slowing of the respiratory rhythm contributes to the soothing of our cardiovascular system and our neuromuscular tensions. It also curbs the production of free radicals, which, when present in excess, attack our tissues.

↦ The Delta Breathing regimen also helps us manage stress and negative emotions, especially the fear connected to illness. As soon as an illness is announced, Delta Breathing is useful because it enables us to better control the anxiety provoked by this destabilizing news.

↦ You can practice Delta Breathing (almost) anywhere, in all circumstances and positions. The recommended postures are seated (in the coachman position) or lying down.

✦ You must always breathe through the nose (except for a few very particular instances) to filter out pollutants, humidify the lungs, and remove the larger particles of dust and pollution.

✦ The effort must be directed at lengthening the exhalation, never the inhalation, in order to promote gaseous exchanges and eliminate toxins from the lungs.

✦ Learning the complete Delta Breathing technique takes place over five steps that last ten days each: first rhythm control, then abdominal breathing, then pauses with lungs full (then lungs empty), followed by neuromuscular reprogramming exercises, and, finally, pinched-lips exhalation.

✦ You must never fast-forward through the steps. The goal isn't to arrive at the last step as quickly as possible but to reharmonize the metabolism by way of breathing. For this, you must practice progressively and regularly. In order to remain patient, remember this: the first positive benefits are felt on the third day of practice.

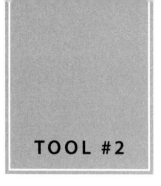

TOOL #2

DELTA NUTRITION

Food is not food if it no longer possesses the power to heal the body. It is only food in word, but not in deed.

HIPPOCRATES, THE ANCIENT FATHER
OF WESTERN MEDICINE

It's been more than twelve years since the World Cancer Research Fund International concluded that a more healthy, balanced diet would result in 100,000 fewer cases of cancer in France. Many doctors share this opinion, including Dr. Laurent Chevallier, a nutritional consultant and attaché to the major teaching hospital Le Centre Hospitalier Universitaire in Montpellier. "Each year in France," he says, "eating junk food causes three times as many deaths as smoking and fifty times more deaths than road accidents. It is, in part, responsible for 30 percent of the cases of cancer, 500,000 cases of heart failure, two million diabetic patients and the eight million obese individuals. Unbelievable! I'm sounding the alarm because during my consultations I am confronted every day with victims of bad eating habits."*

This position was recently confirmed in 2008 by conclusions from the largest international scientific summary, which outlines the

---

*Cited in an article titled "La liste noire de la malbouffe" ("The Junk Food Blacklist") in *Le Point* (March 19, 2009).

connections between nutrition and cancer and is based on more than seven thousand studies. Its figures are alarming: according to the World Health Organization, if no preventive measures are taken, cancer, the number-one cause of death in the world, will lead to 84 million deaths a year by 2015.

These numbers may seem brutal, but they are nonetheless indispensable to underscoring the importance of good nutrition to disease prevention and healing.

After controlled practice of the breath, a second daily act lets us remain alive—nourishment. If we don't eat, we will waste away and disappear, molecule by molecule, tissue by tissue. This may seem obvious, but this point masks a more serious, subtle reality. Contrary to the popular cliché, food doesn't play the same role as the gas we put in our car. It's our source of energy, of course, but it is much more than that. Eating a sufficient quantity of food to stay alive isn't enough; we must eat a sufficient *quality.*

Depending on how we choose and combine them, foods can become promoters of illness. But, luckily, the opposite is also true: our nutritional choices can play an essential role in our return to well-being and health. This is where Delta Nutrition comes into play.

EATING WELL: AN ANCESTRAL KNOWLEDGE THAT WE'VE LOST

Over the course of the past several decades, science has pierced almost all the molecular secrets of foods and the inner workings of digestive physiology. We now know about the essential nutrients: the macronutrients (carbohydrates, fats, proteins, fiber) and the essential micronutrients (vitamins, minerals, trace elements, amino acids, fatty acids, enzymes). We are also now learning what they become within our bodies after we have ingested them.

Nevertheless, this knowledge doesn't stop a good half of the three billion individuals in industrialized nations from being sick from their nutritional imbalances, suffering from obesity, diabetes, hypertension, high cholesterol levels, or metabolic syndrome. One of the keys to resolving these problems lies in how we behave when we face illness and how we think about our health: we need to talk about nutrition, rather than making matters worse by mindlessly eating and generating more imbalance in our system and in our life. In this way we will learn to "resume the dialogue" with foods, as we have done with our breath. Through this dialogue, established on solid scientific grounds, we'll rediscover and recognize the importance of wise choices, combinations, and nutritional rhythms.

Why learn to eat when we already know how to satisfy our hunger? Simply because a big difference exists between eating when we're hungry and eating consciously—knowing basic nutritional rules—and thus eating for health.

First, you should know that when a person's major centers of cerebral control are disturbed, this often causes irrepressible false hunger: snacking and cravings. (Our brain includes neurons that form ganglia, whose role is to control the major balances of the body, among them the satiety center that controls our appetite.) Never forget that the true nutritional rules for health are millions of years old. They evolved by trial and error, along with the development of human beings. They were transmitted from generation to generation, with women most often in charge of inculcating the rules of good nutrition as part of their maternal functions. But for the past fifty years or more the progressive breakup of the multigenerational family has destroyed this chain of transmission in Western societies. Science and, unfortunately, marketing have taken over this role. But if science has often succeeded at explaining, it doesn't know how to educate. And so we find ourselves alone, without rules, without control, and often without intuition. The only pseudoadvice that we receive today is, in reality, pressure to buy that comes from the world of marketing, which has rushed in to fill this gaping hole, with no competency and no ethics. We're indebted to marketing for two generations of obesity and junk food illnesses. With the current, third generation, obesity and metabolic diseases related to nutrition now appear in childhood. This is one of the hidden dramas at the dawn of this new millennium, equal in scale to all the ecological problems that we face.

EATING AND BREATHING: TWO VITAL, INSEPARABLE NEEDS

Nutrition and respiration are closely related. Working in concert, the two produce energy, without which no organism, as simple as it may be, can remain alive. Whether we're talking about a simple cell or a complex being (a newborn human, for example), the first act of life consists of breathing, of drawing indispensable oxygen from the surrounding air. The second act, which occurs almost simultaneously, consists of eating. Respiration and nutrition are therefore integrally linked in the production of this precious vital energy (the nucleotide ATP, mentioned earlier). Breathing provides the body with one type of sustenance—oxygen—while food brings it another—nutrients.

Even if we view eating and breathing as two totally separate and very different acts (one is conscious, voluntary, and a source of pleasure; the other unconscious, often involuntary and generally without flavor), both are equally indispensable to maintaining life and health. Let's not forget that after taking that first breath and letting out that first cry, the newborn placed on his mother's belly has the immediate reflex to turn toward the breast, seeking nourishment. Deep within the instinct to live, beneath layers of a nascent psyche, these two acts play a prominent role in the same vital drive.

FOOD'S ENERGY

We need energy for each of our movements. This is indisputable. But before that we need it so that our organs can function, our glands can produce their hormones, our tissues can regenerate, and our cells can maintain their shape (their structure) and perform their specific activities. As we saw earlier, this energy is produced in each cell, within a small organic factory called a mitochondrion. Mitochondria (the plural of *mitochondrion*) cannot function normally without access to oxygen and nutrients (in particular, glucose), and they need these in quantity, quality, and precise proportions. Over the course of our lives, we consume, on average, 40 tons of food and 13,200 gallons of water that, combined with 4.2 million gallons of oxygen, permit our cells to produce 60,000 kWh of energy! This represents the electric energy consumed by a hot water tank for a family of four over the course of ten years of continuous functioning. Or, to give a more eco-logically correct illustration, the electric energy produced by the total of solar panels covering a basketball court, functioning continuously for fifty years!

But the role of food doesn't end there; along with the macronu-trients (proteins, fats, carbohydrates, and fiber), there are also essen-tial micronutrients.* Vitamins and trace elements don't provide direct energy. But they contribute to the proper functioning of our metabo-lism by way of the thousands of enzymatic reactions they promote, and they figure in the production and overall use of energy by the body. This is how our bodies distribute and judiciously use the pure energy (ATP) produced by the cellular metabolism.

Thanks to the mix of all these fundamental nutrients, our body can regenerate at a rate of 2.5 million new cells per second (some faster than others). At this pace, within seven years all the matter that constitutes our body is replaced, down to the very last atom. This incredible speed justifies all hopes of regeneration and reprogramming, provided we pro-mote the dietary equilibrium of our terrain.

But this reprogramming of our cells can also generate questions and

---

*Macronutrients are what we call the nutrients whose daily intake is calculated in grams (for example, 70 grams of protein for a man weighing 155 pounds). Micronutrients are the trace elements whose daily intake is defined in milligrams (60 mg of vitamin C; 1 mg of vitamin B_1, etc.).

fears insofar as we deliberately scorn the elementary principles of nutritional health.

NO RESTRICTIVE DIET

Food is definitely the key element in our vital processes. So it is no surprise that, according to the quantity and quality of the nutrition we consume, food plays a role in the maintenance of health or the construction of illness, notably cellular problems. Keep in mind: there's nothing magical about nutrition. With the exception of some metabolic diseases or major allergies, nutrition cannot directly heal anything. But it actively modifies, day by day, the biological constants of our vital terrain. And this influences the equilibrium of our health balance. Delta Nutrition can replace our most flagrant dietary errors with health-nutrition practices, improving the terrain that originally led us to illness.

Delta Nutrition doesn't impose a restrictive, frustrating, complicated diet. It's not difficult to start, and it's not difficult to follow. And it's definitely not about overhauling what you eat from top to bottom. As I emphasized earlier, we hate changing our habits. The body and mind can't stand intense, sudden upheavals. Numerous studies have confirmed this. I'm thinking in particular about one that was carried out in the United States and Germany. A medical team offered a group of cancer patients the possibility of replacing chemotherapy and radiation therapy treatments with a very strict diet that required a complete change in their lifestyle and had to be rigorously followed for six months to be effective.* More than 60 percent of the people refused, preferring chemotherapy and radiation therapy, in spite of the long trail of painful side effects associated with those treatments. Drastically modifying their eating habits just seemed too

---

*Cited in the worldwide bestseller by Dr. Bernie Siegel, *Love, Medicine and Miracles* (HarperCollins, 1988).

difficult. Diets that involve big changes (and, in the long term, social isolation) are not generally well accepted by the mind or the body. Anything that requires the body and mind to change too much isn't effective in the long term.

Let's be clear that we're not talking here about attempting to lose weight,* even if by adopting Delta Nutrition's good habits some people will lose the extra pounds that weigh down the work of the metabolism. But if Delta Nutrition sometimes has a slimming effect for overweight patients, it may have a weight-gain effect for those who need it. This weight adjustment—up or down—is only a secondary positive effect that follows the overall metabolic rebalancing (we will come back to this). The main goal is to rehabilitate your body gently, but profoundly, with the objective of giving a new, positive push to all your healing processes.

For those of you who have led a very imbalanced life on a nutritional level, it would be wise to consult the next chapter (Delta Detoxification) before applying the Delta Nutrition advice. You'll find explanations and advice about how to rid the body of waste and toxins that are slowing down and disturbing your metabolic functions. A liver and kidney draining, based on carefully chosen herbs and other plants, should never be neglected. Delta Nutrition's advice will give even more rapid and observable results once the body has been cleared of these toxins and other internal pollutants.

SCIENTIFIC FACTS, EMPIRICAL WISDOM

The dazzling advances in the domain of nutritional science and micronutrition—the study of the impact of vitamins, trace elements, essential fatty acids, and the like, on health—are sadly associated with a serious loss: we have forgotten some of the instructions that help us

---

*An absurd obsession with weight over the past fifty years has paradoxically led to an obesity epidemic due to the rebound effects of diets (the so-called yo-yo effect).

combine foods to prepare dishes and meals that make sense from a health standpoint. It's as if we have come to know the components of a machine better and better but have misplaced the plans to assemble it and the instruction manual on how to use it.

The nutrients contained in foods resemble Lego pieces; the body uses them to construct what it needs: cells, tissues, hormones, vital liquids, and so on. In the same way that you can construct all sorts of different objects (cars, airplanes, houses, bridges) with Lego pieces, your body develops a wide variety of substances and essential tissues with the same set of nutrients. But to thrive, your body must have access to all the necessary nutrients at the right moment, in the right place, in the right quantities, and combined in a timely way (by following the instruction manual).

In every civilization throughout history, ancestral culinary traditions have inculcated rules and habits that respect these needs, according to the foods available in that culture's environment. But the chains of communication for nutritional knowledge have been broken. We no longer know, in an empirical and instinctive way, how to construct a balanced diet without recourse to science.

We don't need to dive in to advanced nutrition and force ourselves to transform our diet by way of a permanent biochemical experiment. For millennia humans have known how to feed themselves instinctively. Empirical knowledge was gained through trial and error, and this led to adopting a diet as varied as possible. At first humans ate harvested fruits, meat from hunting, and fish that were caught. Then cultivated vegetables and grains were added to the diet, along with meat from raised animals. Nutritional knowledge was passed down from generation to generation through traditional recipes, more and more sophisticated but still well balanced and vital to our health (apart from times of war and serious famine).

Traditional dishes like pot roast, couscous from North Africa, and the dishes of rice, fish, and vegetables that are served throughout Africa and Asia supply varied and balanced nutrition to the diet. As long as they are prepared with wholesome ingredients and cooked without too much fat, they are completely compatible with the maintenance of good health. Another example: In countries where meat is rare, populations have a custom of mixing grains and legumes (wheat and chickpeas in North African countries, rice and lentils in Indian cuisine, corn and red beans in South America). This combination is crucial so that the proteins contained in the plants and vegetables can become complete and compensate for any protein deficiency. The contribution of protein is thus optimized, even in the absence of a regular supply of animal protein.

And these good nutritional habits, found throughout the world, were developed long before humans knew the constituents of their foods and the importance of them in the maintenance of health.*

THE EVOLUTION OF NUTRITIONAL HABITS

So where has this indispensable knowledge gone? We have already emphasized how much the breakup of the extended family in Western countries has disrupted the transmission of culinary habits from generation to generation. Add to this the fact that women, who were once in charge of feeding the family, no longer have enough time to spend on the task because their role in society is no longer limited to caring for the household.

Nowadays information about food abounds, yet our nutritional education is weaker than ever. We eat as if we're applying ourselves to piling up our Lego pieces, but in the most random order, without ever succeeding at building any kind of recognizable, usable object.

Delta Nutrition offers you an effective construction plan so that your food combinations once again make sense. This will help you rediscover the reality of foods, to tame them so they'll again become friends of your body and your health. For more than fifty years our

*We should always build our scientific knowledge on the world's ancestral wisdom.

bodies and foods have been angry with one another and have conducted an ongoing "dispute" (excess weight, metabolic syndrome). It's high time they reconcile these differences! This reconciliation is especially urgent when a person has cancer or another serious disease. The devastation from bad eating lies silent and below the surface. We continue to digest everything, but we certainly don't assimilate everything; therein lies the trap. It takes years before nutritional imbalances tip the life balance over the Delta Point from health to illness. But when someone is diagnosed with a tumor, time is of the essence. Nutritional errors have already weighed so heavily on the sick side of the life balance that symptoms have appeared. It's urgent to help the body change direction by using all means available to awaken our healing abilities.

Another element that has heavily influenced the evolution of our nutritional habits: the endless quest to lose weight. Contemporary society, obsessed by appearances, has generated absurd nutritional behaviors directly related to a compulsive desire to lose weight. Certainly excess weight, and even more so obesity, "weighs" on the bad side of the balance. Losing weight can then play a part in a return to health. But the cult of the image and the drive to slim down at all costs has led weight-loss candidates to seek rapid results by way of extremely restrictive or unbalanced diets, ignoring basic rules of nutrition (for example, high-protein, low-calorie, Atkins, Mayo, and Hollywood diets, to name just a few). Not only do these diets create imbalances and deficiencies that are detrimental to our health, but their results are ephemeral. In the vast majority of cases, people regain the weight they've initially lost, often along with a few additional pounds. This is the famous yo-yo effect. Our health does not benefit from this frenetic search to lose weight, which has nothing to do with our physiology. But good health is completely compatible with the pursuit of an ideal weight, which corresponds to our physiological, biological, and metabolic reality, and not fantasy; in short, to our health.

Delta Nutrition offers a nutritional rebalancing with the goal of reharmonizing the metabolism, both the major functions of assimilation and the construction of the body. All its other possible impacts are just side effects of this overall reharmonization. Those who follow the advice of Delta Nutrition will be surprised at how much better they feel, how much more energy they have, how much better they sleep, and they might even lose a few pounds if they need to (or gain some, if they're too thin). Many elements will directly weigh on the healthy side of their life balance, improving their recuperation and promoting the action of any other necessary treatments

BIG NUTRITIONAL TRANSFORMATIONS

After mentioning the visible part of the nutritional iceberg, we must now take a look at the submerged part—a part less well known, because it is less exploitable on a marketing level and therefore covered less in the media. Over the course of millennia, we humans have progressively modified the way we live and our bodies have always adapted. This gives rise to two key questions: Why do we now have such a complex, maladjusted relationship with food? And why have Western societies seen the appearance of so many metabolic illnesses linked to food (obesity, cardiopathy, diabetes, hypertension)? The answer to both is simple: our way of eating has changed more in the past fifty years than it did over the course of the preceding fifty centuries! Even if we humans proved to be infinitely adaptable over the centuries, so many more upheavals have taken place over just a few decades that our bodies have not had time to adapt. Add to that a basic fact: For the first time in history, these changes affect the actual structure of foods. Refined, stripped of nutrients, lacking vitamins, full of chemical additives and preservatives, many foods have become strangers to our metabolism and our body can barely digest or assimilate them.

The first cause of this transformation is without precedent—globalization. Because of the exponential evolution in modes of transportation and international exchange, any kind of food can be found anywhere on the planet during any season. But that involves treating these foods, modifying them, transforming them so that they can be easily preserved and last longer. This commercial reality and industrial necessity have produced multiple types of treatment: refining, irradiation, added stabilizers and preservatives, and the like. The more food is refined, the simpler its biochemical structure, and the more it is stable, controllable, and easy to preserve. By refining foods, we bet on both sides: we simplify their overall composition, and we make it easier to preserve them. One example is flour. When it's made from whole wheat, it contains fifty-seven different components: carbohydrates, vitamins, minerals, fibers, enzymes, yeasts. After refining, the flour we call *white* contains only a tiny portion of those components. Its composition can be compared to a pure carbohydrate. Of course, the product is a lot more stable, making it easy to keep and transport. But its impact on the metabolism is much more abrupt and violent than that of the basic, whole food.

Refining isn't possible for all types of foods, so the food-processing industry has invented other preservation techniques. Irradiation, for example, consists of exposing certain fresh foods (fruits and vegetables, for the most part) to radiation that slows the action of microorganisms responsible for decomposition over time. Additives* (preservatives, flavor and substance enhancers, artificial colors and flavors) preserve industrialized products longer: prepared dishes, packaged sauces, candies and pastries, and so on. In the end, the nutritional losses due to refining add to the effects of all the industrial processes to give us new types of foods that our bodies have a harder and harder time recognizing and metabolizing

These industrial transformations thus cause major mutations, progressive shifts in our equilibrium and our digestive and assimilating functions. This is one of the main sources of the many contemporary

---

*These additives represent more than 1,500 substances worldwide, of which more than 800 must still be proved harmless and 80 have already been declared toxic in some countries after being widely used for decades.

nutrition-based health problems: multiple allergies, weight issues, pre-diabetes, metabolic syndrome, in addition to destabilizing modifications of our metabolic terrain (notably hyperacidity). These transformed foods enjoy an even greater success in Western countries because they respond perfectly to the evolution of nutritional habits. These days the time devoted to preparing meals is three times less than it was fifty years ago. Resorting to prepared dishes and packaged, precooked foods is therefore inevitable.

Delta Medicine isn't suggesting a return to the eating habits of our ancestors. It simply hopes to inform, educate, and help you make sense of these new foods of our era. Delta Nutrition lets you combine unhealthy foods so that their negative nutritional impact is neutralized, thus sending an overall rebalancing message to the body that promotes all healing processes.

THE CONSEQUENCES
OF DIETARY TRANSFORMATIONS

One of the major consequences of these dietary transformations is the disturbance of a fundamental mechanism: the control of our sugar level. Our blood constantly transports sugar (or, more precisely, glucose) to all the cells that need it for cellular metabolism. But the circulating blood sugar level must remain as stable as possible. This stability is guaranteed by the production of insulin, a major hormone secreted by the pancreas, a digestive organ.

Glucose is principally supplied by foods called carbohydrates. These are sweet foods, of course (white sugar, fruits, candies, jams, pastries), but also numerous savory foods, such as starches (potatoes, beans, lentils), grains, and preparations that contain them (bread, rice, pasta, pizza, quiche). Not all dietary carbohydrates are identical. Those in the first group have a more simple composition, similar to pure glucose, and they travel very quickly through the bloodstream. The others have a more complex composition and must be separated into simpler elements during digestion before entering the bloodstream to be delivered to the cells. Here we touch on a major point: the refining that the majority of grains and starches undergo makes their carbohydrates much more rapidly assimilated by the body. Even if the sweet flavor isn't there on your taste buds, refined foods can behave a lot like pure glucose. And for fifty centuries the human body never had to manage such a "sugary impact" from savory foods. This is one of the hidden causes of modern weight problems.

To measure the impact of carbohydrates on the body, scientists use a simple tool—the glycemic index. This index is expressed by a number between 0 and 100, 0 being the absence of impact and 100 being maximum impact—that of pure glucose. The industrial transformation that grains and their derivatives undergo considerably raises their impact on the glycemic index, sometimes doubling it. A simple example: rice. The grain provided by this herbaceous plant is very rich in carbohydrates. Yet brown rice has a glycemic index of 45 to 55, which means it's a perfectly healthy food, falling into the average glycemic index range. Partly milled rice (that is, partly refined) has a slightly elevated glycemic index of 65. This is still reasonable, and tolerated, by our bodies. But white rice, completely refined, sees its glycemic index climb to 75, and if this rice is precooked, the glycemic index sometimes reaches 90. This in no way changes the caloric density of the rice, but it doubles its digestive impact on the pancreas. It's one of the best-kept secrets of modern "bad food."

While refining modifies the nature of carbohydrates, packaging also plays a role. Cooking and preparation time must be factored in: the longer a food that's high in carbohydrates is cooked, the more quickly it is assimilated by the body and therefore the higher its glycemic index climbs. Carrots, for example, have a reasonable glycemic index if consumed raw (between 45 and 50). This is higher for cooked carrots (70), and more so if they are reduced in a purée (80 to 85). Again, the impact on the pancreas has now doubled. This doesn't mean that cooked carrots are not as good for you as raw carrots. But they ought to be combined differently with other foods to moderate their digestive impact. Our ancestors knew how to do this empirically, by way of traditional recipes, to serve meals for health and vitality.

THE ROLE OF FOOD
IN METABOLIC PROBLEMS

What does it matter, you might say, as long as we digest our food well? Therein lies the problem: we digest it well and assimilate it badly. This is another significant nutritional trap because of how food affects the pancreas. This organ is very important to our bodies, because it largely controls the circulating blood sugar level, which must remain stable, within a range of 0.7 to 1 gram per liter of blood. Below the minimum, the body is at risk of hypoglycemia, manifested by intense fatigue, dizzy spells, or even fainting (and coma if the blood sugar level falls extremely low). Above that range, an individual runs the risk of developing diabetes with severe pathological results (notably eye, vascular, and cerebral complications). So the blood sugar level must be carefully regulated by the major hormone insulin, secreted by the pancreas. When we eat foods with an elevated glycemic index, an influx of sugar rushes abruptly into our blood. And our body and organs hate anything abrupt.

Industrial transformations have made the glycemic index of many foods climb, placing greater and greater strain on our pancreas. The abruptness of these sudden influxes of glucose progressively irritates the pancreas on a biological level and disrupts the age-old precision of its secretions. Little by little, our insulin flow becomes deprogrammed. Not only is the pancreas fatigued, these untimely secretions leave behind an insulin residue, causing a small, temporary hypoglycemic crisis after food is eaten. This slight decrease in the blood sugar level then follows each excessive increase. This phenomenon brings with it a disruption of the pancreas in the long term (sometimes referred to as insulin resistance), associated with chronic fatigue syndrome as well as sleeping and concentration problems.

The brain experiences these hypoglycemic mini-crises as a repeated assault. And it is very sensitive to this. Don't forget that glucose is its main food source, along with oxygen. Any lack is experienced as a form of aggression that leads to a survival conflict. This is the emergency mode, which has a direct impact on the metabolism by secreting adrenaline and serotonin. These reactions can, in the short term, disrupt the production of certain cerebral neurohormones. This leads to an incorrect functioning of our satiety center. Feelings of false hunger surface, pushing a person to eat, even though the body doesn't need food.

This is how multiple transformations in our dietary habits and even in the nature of our foods lie at the root of overeating, as well as chronic fatigue syndrome, sleep disturbances, and depression—all blights of our modern way of life. But they're also responsible for the explosion of metabolic diseases. According to the Centers for Disease Control and Prevention, looking at figures from 2005–2007 and 1995–1997, new cases of diabetes almost doubled in the United States over this ten-year period. Likewise, a study at the Harvard School of Public Health analyzed diabetes data from 1980 to 2008 and found that the number of people with diabetes worldwide has more than doubled. For the first time ever there are more obese people on the planet than there are people suffering from hunger. Thus we can count more than a billion people who are suffering in one way or another from metabolic disorders related to nutritional factors.

Of course, science has come up with numerous medicinal and chemical responses to most of these disorders. There are drug treatments for diabetes, hypertension, and high cholesterol. But with any metabolic disease related to dietary factors, dietary rehabilitation ought to be the first healing tool. It absolutely must accompany any treatments so that they are fully, and above all durably, effective.

THE ROLE OF FOOD IN CANCER

Everything we have just described concerns our overall metabolic equilibrium. All the imbalances we have just talked about weigh heavily on the bad side of our life balance. But that's not all. Food also has a more direct impact on the genesis of cancer.

Beyond weight problems, it is from food that our body builds itself during childhood and adolescence and then regenerates throughout adulthood. The way we feed ourselves exerts an important influence on cellular life and on all its disorders. Numerous studies have shown that foods with a high glycemic index promote the growth of tumors, which need glucose to develop. Added to that is the fact that the secretion of insulin, destined to regulate the blood sugar level in case of an abrupt glycemic rush, is accompanied by a substance called insulin-like growth factor 1, or IGF1, that stimulates tissue growth. All types of cells benefit from it, including cancerous cells that make use of this substance to accelerate their proliferation.

Since the beginning of the twentieth century the consumption of refined sugar has tripled, without taking into account the increase in consumption of industrially derived products (sweets, candies, pastries), and the nearly systematic addition of sugar to most mass-produced dishes. Closely watching the contribution of carbohydrates is therefore a first essential step when a person is affected by a cellular problem. I will soon explain how you can lower the glycemic load of your meals so that you'll give your pancreas a rest without "nourishing" your cancer. You can do this simply, without completely altering your way of eating.

At the same time, it's important to diminish the contribution of proteins, especially during the first weeks that follow the diagnosis of cancer and before any surgical procedure. Of course, the body needs protein to maintain muscle mass and the health of our organs, and also for a number of other functions, including maintaining immunity.

The components of these proteins (amino acids) are indispensable to the brain for producing neurotransmitters, the endocrine glands for secreting hormones, and all the organs for regenerating. I'm not asking you to stop consuming all animal products. But tumors are protein masses that benefit from any contribution that's high in animal proteins (white and red meats, poultry, high-fat and fermented cheese, eggs). This is why it's better to immediately lower your consumption of proteins for three to four weeks as soon as a diagnosis has been made. You won't run any risk of protein deficiency.

The recommended amount is simple to calculate: count a little more than 0.5 gram of protein per 2.2 pounds (1 kg) of body weight. In other words, 35 grams of protein per day for a man weighing 155 pounds, or 27 grams for a 120-pound woman. Choose light proteins (with few saturated fats), such as poultry or fish. It is also imperative to sharply decrease all fats from the diet during these three to four weeks, because they promote inflammation of the tissues.

THE RULES OF DELTA NUTRITION

In the face of this rapid nutritional evolution, with little respect for our well-being, we must all renew a healthy relationship with food, but for those affected by a cellular problem, this is especially crucial. We must reestablish efficient, respectful communication between food, our body, our metabolism, and our brain. This is what Delta Nutrition offers.

Before delving in to the details of practical applications, there remains one aspect of the problem to discuss. All dietary rehabilitation, no matter how minor, involves change. And, as explained earlier, humans are resistant to abrupt changes. This is why the advice I'm going to give you doesn't require any drastic changes. The only effort that I ask of you is to make a decision. Decide to take your healing into your own hands. Decide to reprogram the major equilibriums (biological and nervous) of your body. Delta Nutrition only requires you to develop a bit of the curiosity and motivation indispensable to understanding what's going on in your body.

Understand that the mini-crises of residual hypoglycemia that follow the haphazard secretions of insulin provoked by modern diets interfere with the production of certain cerebral neurohormones (notably serotonin). But these neurohormones are not just content with coloring our mood and state of mind; they also affect the satiety center that makes us stop eating when our body has received enough food. By following the advice below, you will progressively restore full functioning of your satiety center. Then it will be that much easier to regulate your food intake. The key to your new dietary habits doesn't lie in deprivation and frustration but in a serene and calm relationship with food that you are going to build.

You don't have to become a dietitian or go shopping and prepare meals with a calculator in hand. But you can—you must—become enlightened, endowed with the practical knowledge that will allow you to fully participate in your own healing.

Even if it might seem trivial, I find the example of a car to be a vivid one: when you have a problem with the radiator and your car overheats, simply knowing that you shouldn't sit too long in traffic jams or climb narrow mountain roads that demand a lot from your motor can be enough to avoid a breakdown. This doesn't make you a well-informed mechanic. This doesn't repair your radiator. But it does limit the consequences of the problem, and it gives you time to reach the nearest garage, where a specialist is waiting for you. The relationship that you maintain with your body arises from the same kind of mechanism: you will become a more active agent in your healing if you acquire this understanding and if you reconcile yourself to what the modern diet has become after fifty years of uncontrolled (and, unfortunately, uncontrollable) technological transformations.

THE METABOLIC INDEX:
THE BASIS OF METABOLIC RESTORATION

Sure, you say, but how do we begin? How do we catch up on this fifty-year rupture with ancestral empirical knowledge? It would be illusory to try to return to the foods and dietetic rules of our great-grandparents. And it would be equally useless to dream of turning in to a nutritionist with the wave of a magic wand.

In order to help you, I have worked in conjunction with a medical team at the University of Tokyo in Japan to develop a new dietary index that integrates the glycemic index of all foods (their impact on the pancreas and the resulting insulin secretion), as well as their enzymatic index (how each food is digested and assimilated), and, in small measure, their caloric index. This comprehensive metabolic index (expressed between 0 and 100) takes into account the overall metabolic impact of foods, allowing you to easily be aware of the weight you place on the healthy side or on the sick side of your life balance. It's called the Metabolic Index.* From there we have classified foods into three major categories based on their ranking in the Metabolic Index.

- Foods in the green category have the lowest Metabolic Index (between 0 and 45); they're beneficial to your metabolic equilibrium.
- Foods in the orange category have an average Metabolic Index (between 45 and 60) and are neutral from a metabolic point of view.
- Foods in the red category have an elevated Metabolic Index, causing the body to deviate from metabolic neutrality and weighing down on the sick side of the balance.

---

*This index is also referred to as the Slim-Data Index.

I would like to emphasize right off the bat that red foods are not forbidden. Just keep in mind that they need to be combined with the same quantity of green foods in order to neutralize the metabolic impact of the red foods. Therefore, any meal is possible: the key term in Delta Nutrition is *health combinations,* because these combinations deliver balancing metabolic messages to the body.

Added to this are a few foods classified separately in the purple zone. These foods either have a very high Metabolic Index or strong toxicity for our digestive and cellular equilibrium. They are *non-foods* in the sense that they deliver very few usable nutrients, but a lot of extremely refined carbohydrates or harmful additives, or both. Potatoes are good food; so is salmon. But mass-produced, smoked salmon-flavor chips are nothing but a molecular heap of foods and synthetic flavors, an insult to both the original foods and to your health.

Foods in the purple zone must be avoided, even by those in good health, and all the more so when you are suffering from a cellular problem. Relatively few foods are listed here.

All the other foods (hundreds of others) are yours to eat. The only stipulation is to combine foods in a way that the overall Metabolic Index of your meals remains within the limits of what your metabolism can easily manage, digest, and assimilate: green for the first few weeks to intensify the balancing messages, followed by orange when you reach cruising speed.

All the foods that are followed by the superscript [P] in the tables on the following pages are rich in proteins. At least one of these foods must be integrated into each of your meals, but without ever consuming one gram of protein more than your daily allowance according to weight. (Protein recommendations for those with cancer were provided on page 90; for general protein recommendations, see page 106.)

You will find a simplified version of this table at the beginning of the book, inside the front cover.

GREEN ZONE
Foods Favorable to Overall Metabolic Equilibrium
Consume Liberally

Vegetables

Artichoke (raw or cooked)	Cauliflower (raw or cooked)	Mushrooms (raw or cooked)
Asparagus (raw or cooked)	Celery (raw or cooked)	Radishes (red or black)
	Cucumber	Sorrel
Bean sprouts (raw or cooked)	Eggplant	Spinach (raw or cooked)
Bell pepper (red, yellow, or green, raw or cooked)	Endive (raw or cooked)	
	Fennel (raw or cooked)	Summer squash (raw or cooked)
	Garlic	Swiss chard
Broccoli (raw or cooked)	Green beans (fresh)	Tomatoes (raw or cooked)
Brussels sprouts	Jerusalem artichoke	
	Leeks	Turnips
Cabbage (raw or cooked)	Lettuce	Zucchini (raw or cooked)
Carrots (raw)		

Fresh Fruits

Cherries	Kiwi	Quince
Clementines	Lemon	Tangerines
Cranberries	Lychee	
Grapefruit	Mandarin oranges	

Nuts

Almonds	Hazelnuts	Walnuts

Grains

Oat bran	Rye	Wheat bran

Legumes

Red beans	Tofu[P]

Dairy

Cottage cheese[P]	Fruit yogurt[P]	Plain yogurt[P]
Fat-free cow's milk[P]	Goat's milk[P]	Sheep's milk[P]
Fresh cheeses (cow, goat, and sheep milk)[P]	Goat's milk yogurt[P]	Sheep's milk yogurt[P]
	Plain fromage blanc[P]	

Fish and Crustaceans

Caviar[P]	Mussels[P]	Semifatty fish (fresh anchovies, goatfish, mullet, sardines)[P]
Clams[P]	Octopus[P]	
Crab[P]	Oysters[P]	Surimi[P]
Crawfish[P]	Prawns[P]	Whitefish (hake, halibut, sole)[P]
Fatty fish (tuna, mackerel, herring, eel, fresh salmon)[P]	Scallops[P]	
	Shrimp[P]	
Lobster [P]	Squid[P]	

Meats and Eggs

All red meats (beef, lamb, duck, mutton, etc.)[P]	Ostrich[P]	Rabbit[P]
Egg whites[P]	Poultry (chicken, turkey, guinea fowl, quail)[P]	Veal[P]
Eggs (soft-boiled, hard-boiled, or poached)[P]		

Canned Foods

Green beans	Plain crab in water[P]	Plain shrimp in water[P]
Hearts of palm	Plain salmon in water[P]	Plain tuna in water[P]

Condiments and Spices

Fresh herbs (basil, chives, coriander, dill, etc.)	Spices (cumin, ginger, curry, pepper, etc.)

GREEN ZONE (continued)
Foods Favorable to Overall Metabolic Equilibrium
Consume Liberally

Desserts

None

Beverages

Black and herbal tea without sugar

Noncarbonated mineral water

Dishes

Beef stew (homemade, with no carrots or potatoes)[P]

Bouillabaisse[P]

Burgers (hamburgers or turkey burgers *of good quality*; not those of the mass-produced, deep-fried variety)[P]

Chicken broth

Coleslaw

Corned beef[P]

Crudités (raw seasonal vegetables in a light sauce)

Egg drop soup[P]

Eggplant parmigiana

Miso soup

Omelets[P]

Roast beef [P]

Roast turkey[P]

Salads (raw seasonal vegetables in a light dressing or vinaigrette)

Soups (made with fresh vegetables, but no carrots or potatoes)

Steak

Steamed mixed diced vegetables

Steamed whitefish[P]

Stuffed cabbage

ORANGE ZONE
Foods Neutral to Overall Metabolic Equilibrium
*Consume liberally, but, in general,
combine these with foods from the green zone.*

Vegetables

Avocado	Okra	Peas (fresh)
Beans (fresh or cooked)	Onion (cooked)	Sauerkraut
Beets (cooked)	Parsnips	Shallots (cooked)
Carrots (cooked)		

Fresh Fruit

Apples (raw)	Mango	Pineapple
Bananas, barely ripe	Melon	Plums
Blackberries	Nectarines	Pomegranate
Blackcurrants	Papaya	Raspberries
Blueberries	Passion fruit	Red currant
Grapes	Peaches	Rhubarb
Guava	Pears	Strawberries
Kumquat	Persimmons	Watermelon

Nuts and Dried Fruit

Brazil nuts	Pecans	Pistachios
Cashews	Pine nuts	Raisins

Grains

Barley	Couscous (by itself)	Rye
Bran bread	Flours (buckwheat, wheat, fine semolina)	Rye bread
Breakfast cereals without sugar or fat (like All-Bran)	Multigrain bread	Sourdough breads (preferably whole wheat or whole grain)
Brown rice (cooked al dente)	Pastas (preferably whole grain, cooked al dente)	Spelt wheat flakes
Bulgur		

ORANGE ZONE (continued)
Foods Neutral to Overall Metabolic Equilibrium
Consume liberally, but, in general,
combine these with foods from the green zone.

Legumes

Broadbeans (fresh or dried)	Lentils	Navy beans
Chickpeas (fresh or dried)	Lima beans (fresh or dried)	Yams

Dairy

Cream cheese	Fat-free cow's milk cheese[P]	Fromage blanc with fruits or herbs[P]
Cooked cheeses (emmenthal, gruyère, etc.)[P]		

Fish and Crustaceans

Breaded fish, well drained after cooking[P]	Salmon roe[P]	Trout roe[P]

Meats and Eggs

Offal (liver, heart, tripe, tongue, sweetbreads, kidneys)[P]	Trimmed and sliced ham[P]	Wild game (venison, etc.)[P]

Canned Foods

Anchovies in salt (rinsed well)[P]	Corn	Pineapple
Chickpeas	Green peas	Sardines in tomato sauce[P]

Condiments

Bouillon cubes (without glutamate)	Natural soy sauce or tamari	Tomato sauce
Green olives	Pickled vegetables	Vanilla in the pod
Mustard (without additives)		

Desserts

Cheesecake

Frozen yogurt

Pies (homemade)

Plain pancakes (no syrup or jam; agave nectar is okay)

Plain waffle (no syrup or jam; agave nectar is okay)

Rice pudding (homemade— very lightly sweetened with unrefined sugar or fructose)[P]

Sorbet

Unsweetened fruit milk shake

Yogurt smoothies

Beverages

Carbonated mineral water

Coffee without sugar

Flavored mineral water without sugar

Fresh orange juice

Red wine (good quality—I glass per meal, diluted with water)

Tomato juice

Vegetable juice

Dishes

Applesauce (without sugar)

Baked beans

Beef and onion panini[P]

Breaded fish with fresh spinach

Buckwheat pancakes

Cannelloni

Chicken and mozzarella panini[P]

Chicken and vegetable sandwich[P]

Shish kebab

Fried chicken[P]

Fried fish[P]

Guacamole

Macaroni and cheese

Moussaka[P]

Tabouli

Nachos (homemade)

Pasta cooked al dente with vegetables

Pastrami[P]

Pork and beans[P]

Ratatouille

Spring rolls

Tacos

Tomato and mozzarella panini

Tortillas

Tuna and vegetable sandwich[P]

Tuna salad[P]

Turkey wrap[P]

Veal parmigiana[P]

Veggie wrap

Wonton soup

RED ZONE
Foods That Threaten the Overall Metabolic Equilibrium
Always combine with foods from the green zone.

Vegetables

Carrot purée

Pumpkin

Vegetable purée

Vegetable soup with potatoes

Winter squash (acorn, butternut, delicata, hubbard, etc.)

Fresh Fruit

Apples (cooked)

Apricots

Bananas (ripe)

Chestnuts

Figs

Nuts and Dried Fruits

Almond paste

Apricots

Dates

Figs

Peanuts (plain)

Prunes

Grains

Bagels

Biscotti (whole grain, unsweetened)

Breads (brioche, challah, French, Italian, rustic French, unleavened, white, whole wheat)

Couscous (precooked)

Crackers (whole grain)

Muesli

Oatmeal

Phyllo dough (cooked in the oven or fried)

Polenta (semolina, cornmeal, or chestnut flour)

Popcorn

Pretzels

Puffed rice pudding

Rice sheets (for spring rolls)

Wheat (precooked)

White rice

Legumes and Starches

Millet

Peas

Potatoes (boiled in water, mashed, fried)

Sweet potato

Dairy

Aged cheeses (camembert, blue, etc.)[P]

Cheese spread (cheddar, port wine, etc.)[P]

Whole cow's milk[P]

Meat and Eggs

Bacon[P]

Cured ham[P]

Fried eggs[P]

Meat loaf[P]

Pork[P]

Sausages (traditional, good quality)

Scrambled eggs[P]

Canned Foods

Anchovies in oil[P]

Fruit in syrup

Herring in oil[P]

Lentils

Navy beans

Sardines in oil[P]

Smoked fish (salmon, whitefish)[P]

Tapenade

Tuna in oil[P]

Condiments

Black olives

Bouillon cubes (with glutamate)

Bread crumbs

Honey

Ketchup (good quality, without additives)

Peanut butter (natural)

Red and white wine ($\frac{1}{2}$ glass, for preparing a dish)

Sweetened, flavored mustard

Vinegar

Desserts

Apple crisp

Brownie

Chocolate (bar, dark, milk)

Chocolate suicide cake

Crème brûlée

Doughnut (homemade)

Flan (homemade—lightly sweetened with unrefined sugar or fructose)[P]

Flan (mass-produced)[P]

Fruitcake

Gingerbreads, spice cakes

Ice cream (without preservatives)

Ice cream cake roll (without preservatives)

Jam

Jell-O

Madeleines

Maple syrup

Milk shake

Muffins

Nutella

Pancakes with sugar, jam, or real maple syrup

Pastries

Pies (mass-produced)

Puddings and creams[P]

Rice cakes (homemade)

RED ZONE (continued)
Foods That Threaten the Overall Metabolic Equilibrium
Always combine with foods from the green zone.

Desserts (continued)

Sugar (brown, raw)

Tiramisù

Turkish delight

Waffle with whipped cream, sugar, or jam

Whipped cream

Beverages

Black or herbal teas (sweetened)

Cappuccino

Champagne

Coffee (sweetened)

Dry alcohols made from grains (whiskey, vodka)

Fruit juice (fresh or mass-produced)

Instant hot chocolate (made with water or milk)

Mineral water (flavored and sweetened)

Red or white wine (good quality)

Dishes

Carrot purée

Carrots sautéed in garlic and parsley

Cheese soufflé[P]

Cheese and bacon panini or sandwich[P]

French toast

Grilled cheese sandwich[P]

Ham and cheese panini[P]

Ham sandwich[P]

Hot dog (good quality only)[P]

Mashed potatoes

Knishes (potato, spinach, kasha, sweet potato; baked or fried)

Macaroni/pasta salad

Pizza

Potatoes au gratin

Potato salad

Pasta al dente in carbonara sauce (traditional recipe)[P]

Puff pastry appetizers

Quiche lorraine (traditional recipe)[P]

Ravioli

Sauerkraut with sausage (traditional recipe)[P]

Sausage sandwich[P]

Three-cheese panini[P]

Tropical fruit salad (bananas, mangos, papayas)

Vietnamese spring roll

PURPLE ZONE
Antihealth and Antivitality Foods
To be avoided (do not eat more than once or twice a week).
No need to combine with green zone foods;
purple zone foods are impossible to rebalance.
They are just bad for your health.

Nuts

Peanuts (flavored)	Smoked and salted almonds

Grains

Chemically flavored crackers	Sweet rolls
Mass-produced pastries	Sweetened cornflakes
Mass-produced white bread	Sweetened, refined, mass-produced breakfast cereals
Precooked pasta	
Precooked white rice	White crackers
Rice puffs	White-flour cookies and biscuits

Legumes and starches

Chips: flavored, smoked, or plain	Dehydrated mashed potatoes

Meats and Eggs

Mass-produced hot dogs, sausages, and lunch meats

Condiments

Chemically processed bouillon cubes	Mass-produced sauces (with preservatives, colors, sugar, and glutamate)
Hot-pressed oils	
Hydrogenated oils and fats	Palm oils
Ketchup (with preservatives and sugars)	Peanut butter (with additives)
Margarine	Soy sauce (with preservatives and additives)
	White sugar

Desserts

Chemically processed, mass-produced candies	Mass-produced cakes
Ice cream (with preservatives)	

PURPLE ZONE (continued)
Antihealth and Antivitality Foods

To be avoided (do not eat more than once or twice a week).
No need to combine with green zone foods;
purple zone foods are impossible to rebalance.
They are just bad for your health.

Beverages	
Apéritifs	Mass-produced beer
Cheap wine	Mulled wine
Fruit alcohols	Soda
Fruit syrups (grenadine, etc.)	

- *Nothing* is forbidden. Only the purple zone foods must be avoided when a person is suffering from a cellular problem or a metabolic problem, because these foods weigh too heavily on the bad side of your life balance (they are truly antihealth foods).
- The only thing that you must pay attention to: Make sure that the overall Metabolic Index of your meals doesn't pass the orange zone. You can eat foods from the green and orange zones without any worries.
- On the other hand, if you want to have something from the red zone, you absolutely must combine it with foods from the green zone to lower the overall Metabolic Index of your nutritional intake.

It's as simple, but as essential, as that.

THE ACID-ALKALINE EQUILIBRIUM

Consider regularly consulting the Acid/Alkaline foods table inside the book's back cover.

In the previous chapter, on Delta Breathing, we saw how the modern diet promotes a progressive acidification of our internal environment. This slight daily increase in acidity contributes to the appearance of numerous imbalances in our biological terrain, which paves the way for cancers and degenerative diseases. This subacidity is due, in part, to the transformation of foods. The refining of grains increases their potential acidification. The increase in our consumption of sugar, fat, and meat compounds this deleterious trend. Age-old good sense teaches us that nature gives with one hand what she can take with the other. Food, which is in large part responsible for this internal imbalance, can become your principal ally in neutralizing it. I'm not going to get into the details of what is called the acid-alkaline equilibrium.* What you need to know is this: all fruits and vegetables are alkalizing overall, even those with a tart or acidic flavor, like lemon, kiwi, orange, and the like. They naturally oppose the excess acidification of our internal environment. Therefore, give them first priority on your menu each day. For salad dressings, use cider vinegar or lemon juice; their organic acids become alkalizing upon contact with gastric secretions. Avoid regularly eating sausages and other prepared meats, refined cheeses with a high fat content, and red meat; digesting them produces a number of acidifying substances. Replace them as often as possible with poultry or fish. Finally, eat whole grains (or semiwhole grains) and limit your consumption of white sugar and sweets.

You can ensure the acid-alkaline equilibrium in your diet by consuming a daily dietary ration of 70 percent alkalizing foods and 30 percent acidifying foods.

As you can see, respecting the Metabolic Index and incorporating health-producing behaviors in your daily life will help you avoid excess interior acidity. A practical and coherent program awaits you; in just two short weeks this health tool will become a true health reflex.

---

*See the excellent book on this subject by Dr. Christopher Vasey, *Acid–Alkaline Diet for Optimum Health* (Rochester, Vt.: Healing Arts Press, 2006).

YOUR DELTA NUTRITION PROGRAM IN PRACTICE

To reprogram your metabolism gently and bring your life balance back to the Delta Point, and tipping toward the side of health, adopt the following program as quickly as possible. It doesn't demand much effort, and you will feel the beneficial effects within just two weeks.

One point to keep in mind: When we talk about a food (or, as seen in some places, a dish), we will refer to a "food unit" or a medium-size portion (this can vary according to your size, gender, age, appetite, and habits). In the context of Delta Nutrition, it's not so much the quantity that counts as the balance between the categories of foods (green, orange, and red).

▲ During the First Two Weeks

■ Concentrate your efforts on an eating regimen that's low on the Metabolic Index by selecting green or orange zone foods for your meals.

■ Include at least one food from the green zone at each meal.

■ Avoid (only during these first two weeks) red zone foods; you will integrate them into your diet later on.

■ Use one of the following food zone combinations during a meal:

I green + I green + I green
I green + I green + I orange
I green + I orange + I orange

■ You should also monitor your acid-alkaline equilibrium ($^1/_3$ acids for $^2/_3$ alkalines) by consulting the chart inside the back cover. Give top priority to vegetables (if you can, 50 percent vegetables that grow aboveground and 50 percent vegetables that grow in the ground), fruits, and herbs.

■ And don't forget to monitor your intake of animal proteins: not more than I gram per 2.2 pounds (I kg) of your weight, or 70 grams for a person weighing 155 pounds, which corresponds to about 140 grams of cooked steak or chicken, 200 grams of fish, or two eggs. Your health depends on it!

Note: If you have cancer, you must limit your intake of proteins even further. See "The Role of Food in Cancer" on pages 89–90. And whatever illness you might have, try to give priority to vegetable proteins or light animal proteins (all fish, preferably fatty fish).

▲ During the Following Two Weeks

■ Progressively integrate foods belonging to the red category, always combining them with green zone foods during the same meal in order to lower the overall Metabolic Index of your food intake.

■ Use one of the following combinations during the course of a meal:

I green + I green + I green

I green + I green + I orange

I green + I orange + I orange

I green + I green + I red

I green + I orange + I red

■ Keep paying attention to your acid-alkaline equilibrium.

■ Continue to monitor your regular but very moderate intake of high-protein foods.

▲ After the First Month

■ Your metabolism has begun to reharmonize. You must now stabilize and anchor this improvement.

■ Continue to avoid antihealth foods in the purple category (not more than twice a month at the very most, if you are irreparably hooked). Continue to combine the red zone foods with green zone foods, in equal quantities, in order to lower the overall metabolic impact of your meal.

■ Always remember to include enough vegetables, fruits, herbs, and spices in order to neutralize excess internal acidity (see the chart inside the back cover).

■ Continue to avoid foods that are refined or contain chemical additives; they are always acidifying.

■ Two or three times a week you can include a supplementary combination to your meals. These are now the combinations available to you:

1 green + 1 green + 1 green

1 green + 1 green + 1 orange

1 green + 1 orange + 1 orange

1 green + 1 green + 1 red

1 green + 1 orange + 1 red

1 green + 1 red + 1 red

DON'T FORGET TO CHEW!

This isn't advice for children in a hurry to go back out and play! It's a basic rule for all adults concerned with reclaiming control of their health. In Delta Medicine, the way you eat matters almost as much as your choice of foods. *Chew well to heal well* is the maxim of all traditional doctors.

Try within reason to consume all your meals in a calm atmosphere, because stress and nervous tension have an aggravating impact on metabolic imbalances related to food. And, above all, take the time to chew well. It's essential for the improvement of your state of health and for your healing.

The slogan *The better you chew, the better you heal!* hangs at the entrance to some clinics that specialize in supporting cancer patients. It's neither about meditating on your food, nor fastidiously counting the number of times your jaw moves, as some extreme Eastern diets suggest.* I'm just asking you to relax, take your time, and not swallow your food whole. A meal should take at least thirty minutes, ideally forty-five. If you have finished eating within only ten minutes, either you haven't chewed enough or your meal is very imbalanced.

Keep in mind: I'm talking about thirty minutes of *chewing*, not thirty minutes of conversation sprinkled with a few minutes of barely chewing because you're not paying any attention to your meal and your mind is focused elsewhere (discussion, television, telephone).

Why insist so much on mastication? First, it reduces food to mush,

---

*These age-old dietary techniques are of inestimable value. But their advice is often delivered in terms of promoting meditation or prayer. This isn't what we are talking about.

which creates closer contact between your alimentary bolus (the name given to a meal once it has passed through the mouth and landed in the stomach) and the walls of your stomach. This facilitates assimilation of the nutrients contained in food. Plus, the longer you chew, the more foods are mixed with saliva. Saliva is an extremely alkalizing substance that balances acids susceptible to developing during the different stages of digestion. The better you prepare your food for digestion by chewing well, the more digestive energy—and therefore healing energy—you derive from that food. The more serious your cellular problem, the longer and more carefully you must chew.

Mastication also causes repeated movements of the jawbone. These movements produce a kind of antistress facial massage, sending calming waves to the brain.

Finally, the act of chewing facilitates the first steps of digestion, lessens the work required of the stomach, and limits the quantity of blood needed to furnish energy to this organ. When we suffer from a cellular problem, whatever it may be, our organic energies are weakened. We must therefore carefully plan in order to create sufficient reserves to awaken and nourish all our healing energies.

SOME ADDITIONAL VALUABLE ADVICE

Beyond the general health and nutrition advice, some foods merit a few more explanations.

Bread

For centuries in France (and in some other European countries as well), bread has constituted one of the foundations of nutrition. At least this was the case until the curse of the dieting madness afflicted the Continent. It's unfair, because good bread is an excellent food, completely compatible with a healthy diet as long as you know how to choose it. To summarize roughly: Good bread is good for your health, bad bread is bad for your health. It's best to choose a semi-whole-grain sourdough loaf. (One hundred percent whole-grain bread may be too dense and difficult for someone with a weakened or imbalanced body to digest.) Sourdough, once regularly used to make dough rise, contains natural bacteria that don't just add air to the bread dough and produce a soft inside. They predigest certain substances present in wheat that our bodies have a hard time digesting and assimilating (notably phytic acid). Chemical yeast, which is frequently used in place of sourdough, produces an artificial aeration of the dough and doesn't act on any of the substances that must pass through a fermentation phase. Paradoxically, white bread made with yeast is digested much more rapidly and easily: it therefore seems light and better for your health. This is a trick that we all can fall for if we don't take the time to learn a bit about nutrition. There's a big difference between speed of digestion and ease of assimilation. Unfortunately, just because it feels easy on your system doesn't make it so! Digested more rapidly, refined carbohydrate nutrients move into the bloodstream quickly, and this produces a strong, irritating impact on your all-important pancreas in the long term. White bread is also more acidifying. All this disrupts the assimilation of the other foods absorbed during the same meal.

I recommend eating partially whole-grain bread because whole wheat can prove to be an irritant for the intestines if you aren't used to it. Partially whole-grain sourdough is a terrific alternative to white bread (which must absolutely be avoided). The former has an average Metabolic Index (about 55), while the latter is very high (up to 90), and this contributes to hypoglycemic attacks, false hunger, tissue acidity, and an overall weakening of our biological terrain. White sourdough bread is not quite as bad, but it's far from ideal. I can't tell you how to find good bread near you, made by a competent, conscientious baker, but more and more bakers are concentrating on making healthy loaves. Professional consciences are awakening.

One last remark: People tend not to consider bread a true food, but rather a sort of accompaniment that is consumed as an adjunct to a meal. This is a mistake. Bread is a food unto itself. When you integrate it into your meal (two nice slices), it constitutes one portion of grains (it is then a dietary unit from the orange category). Think about this when you plan your meals.

Soy Products

This is a vast subject, closely linked to the dictates of food industry marketing. Some people wishing to return to a more natural diet or to prevent high cholesterol levels consume soy derivatives in place of dairy products:* soy milk, soy yogurt, and the like. In reality, these designations are fallacious, because their composition doesn't compare at all to dairy products.† Soy milk or soy yogurt cannot replace dairy products from a nutritional standpoint, because the composition is totally different. Their amino acids (base constituents of proteins) are incomplete and badly divided; in the short term they can cause imbalances of the intestinal flora. Moreover, many people have a hard time digesting and assimilating these types of foods that, quickly digested, can cause diarrhea and flatulence.

In and of itself, soy is a respectable food. But traditionally in Asia it is fermented (tofu, soy sauce, miso). Why? Because, like wheat, it contains substances that are difficult for our body to metabolize. Fermentation helps predigest them, rendering them more easily absorbed. To obtain soy milk, a soybean maceration is mixed and filtered: the result is a thick, whitish liquid. As for what are called soy yogurts, their preparation calls for a number of chemical additives, such as thickeners and texturizing agents. So if you really want to consume soy, choose traditional products, in particular tofu, which is an excellent protein to accompany grains, soups, vegetables, and fish.

---

*"Soy mania" is an American obsession: the United States is the first non-Asian country where the consumption of soy has "exploded." This craze has begun to win over Europe as well, propelled by marketing specialists with no clear understanding of its nutritional implications and the lethargy of the scientific community.
†Still, it must be emphasized that when recuperating from a serious illness, it is essential to limit high-fat dairy products (refined cheeses and whole milk), which are acidifying and allergenic.

Organic Food

Organic foods are clearly of ideal nutritional quality and beneficial for those who have access to them. They're rich in essential nutrients and contain fewer contaminants (see the chapter on Delta Detoxification, Tool #3), and these are two truly important health benefits. Nevertheless, consuming organic foods in no way changes the balance or imbalance of the ingredients in your meals. The nutritional ideal resides in food that is organic *and* balanced, that respects the Metabolic Index and the advice aimed at neutralizing the excess acidity of your internal environment. Under these conditions, I am 100 percent for organic food. The label *organic* has to do with the quality of the food itself, but it has no impact on the more or less balanced use of these products. To return to the image that I evoked earlier, Lego pieces of gold would be beautiful and valuable, but you'd construct an ugly or useless object if you didn't follow the directions (or, worse, if you lost the instruction manual).

Therefore, I generally advise my patients to focus on understanding the nature of foods before anything else. I prefer they begin, first and foremost, by taking control of their meals and internal equilibrium. Then, once this step has been integrated into their daily life, they can, if they want and have the means, choose organic products. Of course, people who are already in the habit of eating organic should continue to do so. Their metabolic rebalancing will be that much more rapid and successful.

But don't forget that you can rebalance your internal equilibrium even if you never have access to organic food. You just need to closely follow the advice given in the following chapter on Delta Detoxification.

USING NUTRITIONAL SUPPLEMENTS CORRECTLY

Many patients ask me, "Doctor, can I take dietary supplements?" My answer is an enthusiastic "Yes!" I've already demonstrated that supplements (outside of exaggerated claims generated by publicity and marketing) are a response to the nutritional deficiencies in our contemporary Western diet and are adapted to the demands and rhythms of our lives today. These products contain essential nutrients and can compensate for the nutritional losses that come from the radical transformation of modern foods. Refining foods results in a serious loss of vitamins, trace elements, mineral salts, and fiber. Industrial agriculture is also partly responsible for this loss, as are certain types of packaging. So supplements make good sense: because our foods are depleted, let's replace this loss with vitamins and supplements. But we should respect a few specific rules if we don't want our good intentions to turn against us.

- Dietary supplements are only useful when carefully chosen, aimed at the needs of the person, and taken in reasonable doses. I am firmly opposed to systematic overdoses. When taken in megadoses or absorbed in too large a quantity, dietary supplements can provoke paradoxical effects, rather than the expected benefits. Instead of protecting the body and facilitating healing, they can lead to an even more rapid downslide into illness. Once again, you should exercise good sense.
- Choose nutritional supplements from natural sources (like seabuckthorn syrup or acerola tablets for vitamin C). Without getting bogged down by useless details, it's worth knowing that synthetic vitamins have a nonliving part that the body must eliminate, and this can cause allergic reactions or paradoxical effects. To return to the example of vitamin C, the scientific name of this vitamin is L-ascorbic acid. But synthetic vitamin C is D-L-ascorbic acid. Because only the L-ascorbic form is usable, the body is forced to eliminate part of this D-ascorbic acid to be able to use it, which fatigues the organs and sometimes causes needless problems.
- On the other hand, when you are dealing with a cellular problem, you must be very careful with certain fat-soluble vitamins, whose surplus is only excreted through urine and remains stocked in

your fat cells. You must especially monitor the intake of vitamin A to avoid any risk of vitamin A overdosing because this would have negative effects on the body. The same applies for certain water-soluble vitamins. It's particularly harmful to overdose on vitamin B_{12} and vitamin B_6—in excess, these B vitamins may promote cancers.

- The advice that I habitually give is simple: always use nutritional supplements made by a reputable laboratory and distributed by pharmacies or reputable health food stores. (Manufacturers that I can personally recommend include Nature's Plus and Solgar.) Choose products that have a more balanced formula and are as natural as possible, including the main vitamins from the vitamin B, vitamin E, and vitamin C families, along with some bioflavonoids (such as citrus extracts). The formulation may also include minerals and trace elements (magnesium, calcium, zinc, selenium). Stay away from products with exaggerated marketing promises. Clear product information is the first guarantee that the manufacturer is reputable.

- Each product is dosed in a specific manner, so you must refer to the manufacturer's directions for the recommended daily allowance.

- A good multivitamin or antioxidant as a three-week treatment with each change of season is generally enough. You should avoid taking dietary supplements continuously so that your body doesn't lose the habit (and ability) to extract all the nutrients it needs from food.

- It's best to take dietary supplements during a meal because by mixing them with food the added nutrients will find the ideal natural environment. That way they are also more easily absorbed by the body, which is, in turn, less fatigued by the action of absorbing them.

- Without intending to vilify the Internet, a revolutionary means of communication, I recommend that you never buy dietary supplements from sites you do not know well. There are numerous fraudulent products sold within the United States as well as in India, China, and Eastern Europe. The pharmaceutical industries in all these countries are not at all suspect, but they unfortunately coexist alongside companies producing counterfeits that are at best ineffective and at worst dangerous to your health.

Thus, *Eat well to heal well* is a slogan that you can (and must) make yours, with the help of your new Delta Nutrition health principles.

Key Points

→ Regularly consult the charts inside the front and back covers of this book.

→ To stay in good health it's not enough to eat a sufficient quantity of food—you must, above all, nourish yourself in sufficient *quality*.

→ Repeated dietary mistakes constitute a major factor in metabolic imbalances and, in combination with other factors, promote cancer, as well as degenerative and autoimmune diseases. Delta Nutrition helps rapidly correct many of these errors.

→ Science is unlocking more and more secrets about foods, but we have forgotten the basic rules and methods that ensure nutritional health and balance.

→ Our foods have changed more in the past fifty years than they have in the past fifty centuries. They're now refined, industrialized, transformed, and full of chemical additives and preservatives. All this explains the explosion in metabolic illnesses related to our diet (obesity, diabetes, metabolic syndrome) and contributes to the increase in the number of cases of cancer diagnosed each year.

→ One of the main consequences of the transformation of our foods is the increase in their sugar impact and their acidifying impact, notably because of the excessive refining of grains and the addition of chemical additives.

→ Studies have shown that a diet with a high glycemic load promotes the growth of tumors; foods too rich in animal proteins have this effect too (because tumors are protein masses).

✦ Delta Nutrition doesn't advise you to go on a diet but rather encourages you to recognize the nutritional basis of foods and nutritional combinations.

✦ Delta Nutrition is based on a new nutritional index, the Metabolic Index, which takes into account the glycemic index of foods (their impact on the pancreas and insulin secretion), the enzymatic index (their impact on digestion and assimilation), and, in small measure, the caloric index.

✦ The foods are classified into three color zones: green (those favorable to overall metabolic equilibrium), orange (those neutral on a metabolic level), and red (those that have an impact that is too strong on the organs, except if combined with green zone foods).

✦ Added to this are a few purple zone foods, true "antifoods," which contribute very little by way of nutrients but a lot in terms of chemical substances.

✦ The principle of Delta Nutrition is to combine foods during the same meal so that the nutritional intake remains within the orange Metabolic Index. This lets us regulate the glycemic contribution without prohibiting any food (aside from a few purple foods, which are considered antihealth).

✦ In cases of cancer, during the first few weeks Delta Nutrition also recommends limiting the consumption of animal proteins, fats, and rapidly assimilated sugars so as not to promote the inflammation of the tumor (all these foods are acidifying and awaken or increase cellular microinflammations).

✦ The principles of Delta Nutrition also integrate the acid-alkaline equilibrium: some foods are acidifying to the body, while others are alkalizing. Excessively consuming acidifying foods makes the biological terrain too acidic, which encourages the development of chronic diseases. In general, sausage, red meat, saturated fats, refined cheeses, and sweets are very acidifying, while fruits, vegetables, seasonings, and spices are alkalizing. You should strongly favor the latter.

✦ You must chew sufficiently in order to engage your digestive forces. This helps to more easily mobilize all your healing forces.

✦ Taking nutritional supplements is advised, as long as you avoid overdosing on certain vitamins (vitamins A, B_6, B_{12}, etc.). You must choose well-balanced nutritional supplements, formulated by a reputable manufacturer, and take them as part of a three-week treatment at the change of each season (during meals to facilitate absorption).

✦ Beware of Internet promises, which may be devoid of ethics, controls, and scruples, relating to supplements. Numerous toxic products on the market put your health at risk.

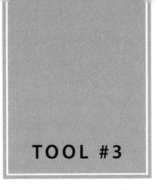

TOOL #3

DELTA DETOXIFICATION

Healing depends on the unobstructed, efficient operation
of all components of the healing system. . . . One of the
greatest threats to the system is toxic overload from the
multitude of harmful substances in today's environment.

DR. ANDREW WEIL,
SPONTANEOUS HEALING

Our cellular, tissue, and organic systems are invaded and attacked daily by numerous kinds of pollution and toxins from the air, food, and, in some cases, medical treatments. But as Dr. Andrew Weil explains in his book *Spontaneous Healing*, "Your body's ability to eliminate unwanted substances depends on the healthy functioning of four systems: the urinary system, the gastrointestinal system, the respiratory system, and the skin. . . . The liver processes most of the foreign chemical compounds, detoxifying them if possible, or breaking them down to simpler compounds that can leave the body via one of those four routes. In order to maintain your eliminative capacity, those four systems must be in good working order." Delta Detoxification is therefore targeted at the liver, the "orchestra conductor" of the body's filtration or detoxification systems.

I have already talked about waste, toxins, and metabolic pollution.

The production of these wastes is a normal and inevitable consequence of cellular life. On the other hand, what is totally avoidable is the accumulation of these residues in our tissues. Luckily, we have very efficient organs that neutralize and eliminate them, and they do their work effectively as long as they aren't overwhelmed by the magnitude of the job.

Two scenarios take place nowadays: either our organs are subjected to a chronic excess of pollution that leads them to become progressively overwhelmed, or these pollutants, although maintained at a "normal" level, cannot be correctly managed because our neutralizing and eliminating organs are compromised. And sometimes (this is most frequently seen in people with cancer), the two scenarios coexist. The best detox techniques must help limit the impact of various wastes and internal and external pollution and also support and cleanse the key organs. This is the twofold goal of Delta Detoxification.

Multiple atmospheric and nutritional contaminants, sedentary living, stress—these all increase the quantity of toxins and wastes that our bodies must handle. Sometimes our organs of elimination need a little help. Several simple, natural techniques can aid them in doing their work. This is what detoxification is, or, to repeat a somewhat trendy expression, this is what a detox program is.

Of all the techniques I recommend in this book, this one is the most talked about in the press. I'd like to take you beyond this media overexposure by helping you understand the scientific processes and metabolic limits of this tool for health that I have used for close to thirty years. As with the other Delta techniques, we are going to draw the best and simplest strategies from various detox plans and programs.

These techniques have been given so much attention by the press, at times accompanied by wildly exaggerated promises, that it has prompted outrage among some leaders at medical schools (and rightly so). They have characterized these programs as useless, emphasizing that the body has all it needs to rid itself of toxins. This is true! Even after a gigantic holiday meal, it only takes the body two or three days to eliminate the excess direct toxins (uric acid, bile salts, saturated fats). But this only takes care of our direct metabolic wastes. The situation is not the same for internal and external pollutants (free radicals, heavy metals, chemical additives in food, electromagnetic radiation). These pollutants are too numerous and too new, and our bodies have no biologically programmed elimination routes for them. For millennia the human body has been infinitely adaptable, but it hasn't had enough time to adjust to these new toxic wastes. They then pollute our filter organs (kidneys, liver, digestive tract) slowly (and inexorably). The Delta Detoxification program's objective is to ease the workload of these key organs and make them function at their maximum "biological power of elimination," so they will, in turn, help support all our healing forces.

THE MAJOR EMUNCTORY ORGANS

To drain, purify, dissolve, neutralize, eliminate, and cleanse in order to heal the body better: this could be the definition of *detoxification*. If this detox program is important for people subject to chronic fatigue or overall ill-being, it is all the more so for cancer patients. Medical treatments for cellular problems are often highly toxic and associated with a number of side effects. They demand increased efforts from the patient's body to assimilate and eliminate wastes (metabolites). The liver, where the major part of medicinal molecules are transformed, deserves some extra support with this weighty task. Science calls our organs of elimination *emunctory*. The main ones are the intestines, the liver, the kidneys, and the lungs. (The Delta Breathing exercises contribute to pulmonary Delta Detoxification.) The skin can also play a role in the elimination of toxins by way of perspiration and even by way of certain chronic cutaneous eruptions.

Before diving in to the practical details of the daily detox exercises, let's spend some time with these organs that are so essential to our internal health equilibrium. Like all living entities, each cell that makes up our body produces waste. These wastes are spewed into the liquid environment in which they are swimming, the so-called interstitial liquid. This liquid is continually drained and regenerated by thousands of small metabolic reactions. One part of the liquid loaded with wastes is regularly excreted via the circulatory and the lymphatic systems. The latter is made up of a network of canals from the bottom of the body to the top. The lymph is a whitish liquid, thick and viscous, that circulates in these lymphatic canals and flows into the circulating venous blood at the level of the clavicles (the collarbones). This simplified explanation allows us to better visualize the inside of the body and its metabolic pathways.

So the venous blood collects the majority of the toxins coming from the metabolic pathways. This blood has two recycling centers: the liver, which filters some of the wastes, and the kidneys, which hold on to the rest. The wastes held in the kidneys are evacuated through urination. Those filtered by the liver are neutralized and transformed inside this treatment center itself, then discharged with the bile in the digestive system. This leads us directly to another very important waste treatment center: the intestines (and their rich bacterial flora). They ensure the evacuation of the large nutritional wastes produced by digestion. A big part of the assimilation of nutrients occurs through the narrow walls of the small intestine. The rest, everything that serves no use (including the wastes discharged by the liver), passes through the colon and is eliminated in the form of excrement.

THE ROLE OF DETOXIFICATION

The detox exercises that I offer are, like all the other Delta Medicine techniques, simple and easy to incorporate into your daily life. They are beneficial for everyone but take on particular importance for people affected by cancer.

Imagine a heating system encrusted with soot: a bad boiler doesn't produce enough heat and uses way too much wood or fuel. If you have it cleaned, its overall functioning will be optimized. Our bodies work the same way. When they're encrusted with internal and external pollution, their overall metabolism is disturbed and slowed down. As long as the life balance leans toward the healthy side, these disturbances go unnoticed. At most they may make the healthy side waver, without actually causing it to cross the Delta Point. But when a cellular problem has been diagnosed, the Delta Point has been crossed and the balance is already leaning to the side of sickness. In this case, the least additional disturbance will weigh heavily.

Moreover, all the other Delta Medicine tools will have that much more effectiveness and impact when the body is relieved of these excess pollutants. Intense medicinal treatments (chemotherapy, long-term corticosteroid therapy) will also work better, and the numerous toxic metabolites that they generate will be more easily transformed into cellular waste and excreted. A number of medicines are made up of chemical molecules that become directly active in the body once they're transformed by the liver. The new molecules that are formed this way are the metabolites of the medicine. The extent of side effects specific to each medicine depends on their degree of toxicity. These side effects are even more significant if our organs are contaminated, or compromised by an inflammatory or allergic reaction. This explains the extreme diversity of side effects observed for the same molecule in different patients.

Delta Breathing (Tool #1) acts as a natural detoxification of the lungs, which themselves play an essential role in the elimination of gaseous waste. So from time to time, try practicing the Delta Breathing exercises in natural surroundings, in an area far from urban pollution (in the forest, in the countryside) to amplify their detox effect even more. Here now are the practical techniques of Delta Detoxification that will help support the work of your brave but exhausted detox organs: your intestines, liver, and kidneys.

▲ Intestinal Detoxification

Talking about intestinal detoxification may seem a bit old-fashioned. But it shouldn't, because correct intestinal functioning is crucial if we want every chance of preventing illness and healing from it.

Regular digestive transit doesn't necessarily mean having a bowel movement every day. We each have our own particular rhythm: for some, this is twice a day, for others, this is once every two days. Once a day is an average, not a norm. The only norm is not to go less than once every two days. These days it's understood that the prolonged contact of fecal matter with the walls of the digestive tract (principally the colon) causes irritation, inflammation, and the localized degeneration of the digestive mucus, which can lead to diverticulitis and certain types of cancer.

To facilitate digestive transit naturally, outside any known intestinal pathology, the most simple acts are the most effective, provided they are practiced regularly.

- Prunes have a reputation as gentle, natural laxatives, and rightfully so. But you must know how to use them so that you avoid any risk of irritation or intolerance. Soak four dried prunes overnight in a glass of water to rehydrate them. The next day, while you are preparing your morning meal, boil them for two to three minutes to soften their fibers, and consume them lukewarm along with your breakfast.

- Think about integrating a daily ration of raw vegetables (chewed well) into your diet. Rich in fiber, they naturally promote digestive transit. For the most part, nutritional fibers are not assimilated by our bodies. They resist the different stages of digestion and arrive in the intestine without being altered. But throughout the entire operation, they absorb some of the water, fats, and toxins they encounter, which causes them to expand. This increases the volume and softness of stools and facilitates evacuation.

- If the above techniques are not enough, add a teaspoon of nutritional fiber found at pharmacies and health food stores to your daily serving of raw vegetables. You can also mix it into applesauce or yogurt and let it expand for three minutes before consuming it. My preferred dietary fibers are oat bran and powdered wheat bran, which don't irritate the intestine and don't fatigue or exhaust the digestive system.

■ You should also think about drinking enough water, in a regular and measured way. This practice is indispensable so that your stools aren't too dry and difficult to evacuate.

I recommend that you add a daily "intestinal timed training" to this basic advice. Behind this somewhat technical term is a simple reality: choose a time of the day when you are sure you won't be bothered, preferably in the morning. Then each day, at the same time, sit down on the toilet for five minutes without doing anything—not even reading. The idea isn't to force but to retrain your intestinal functioning by way of this regularity. You will thus program an evacuation reflex. Be patient and don't obsess over the results. Just be content with focusing your attention on your intestinal functioning without making any effort. The association between this retraining and the small preparatory steps outlined above will overcome the laziest of intestines.

After three weeks at the most, you will obtain lasting results that might be surprising if you have suffered from chronic constipation over the years.

Again, the key to success and effectiveness lies in practicing these small techniques with motivation and regularity. If the advice gives you violent results (more than two stools a day), decrease the doses of prunes and bran until you find the formula that works for you. A too-rapid acceleration of bowel movements can irritate your intestine and results in a loss of essential nutrients. It's a matter of using good sense and finding a happy medium.

▲ Liver Detoxification

As we have said, the liver is the major treatment center for toxic substances. This large organ is found in the abdomen, just below your ribs, on the right side. The consumption of nutritional pollutants (pesticides; residues from chemical fertilizers; artificial colors, flavors, and texture enhancers; preservatives) has increased over the course of the past several decades in an exponential manner. Add to this atmospheric pollutants (part of which pass into the blood during pulmonary exchanges) and residues from the chemical medicines that are absorbed in great quantity by cancer patients because they're an indispensable form of treatment.

All these toxic substances accumulate in the bloodstream at the same time that wastes from our own cellular metabolism arrive. While our vital fluids pass through the liver, they are filtered by this hardworking, efficient organ that retains the wastes and transforms them before getting rid of them. The liver is extremely adaptable, but its adaptability has its limits. Here are some things you can do to keep it from becoming congested and improve its efficiency.

- Black radish is the liver's number-one friend. You can eat it if you like its slightly bitter flavor, but to obtain optimal results as part of the detoxification plan, you'd have to consume it every day, which would quickly become tedious. It's better to use extracts. Choose an aqueous extract (in vials), because the tinctures contain alcohol and are toxic to the liver, even in very small doses. Black radish drains the hepatic toxins and increases the production and evacuation of bile. A black radish treatment must be progressive. If you attempt to detoxify your liver too abruptly, you could cause a sudden toxic discharge that can lead to headaches and nausea. Adopt black radish progressively with this treatment:
  - First take ¹/₂ vial of liquid extract of black radish (*Raphanus sativus*) each morning for one week.
  - Over the course of the following week, take a full vial in the morning; then one vial in the morning and evening for the next seven days.
  - Finally, to end your treatment, return to only one vial in the morning, again for seven days.
- You can do this black radish treatment once every three months (ideally with the change of seasons).
- Some truly valuable medicinal plants complete the action of the black radish, notably artichoke and boldo. They are both choleretic (that is, they activate the production of bile) and cholagogue (meaning they

facilitate the evacuation of bile toward the digestive organs). In phytotherapy it is the leaves of the artichoke that are used and not the flower bud, which is typically consumed as a food. Artichoke leaf tea is very bitter, so I recommend that you consume it instead in vial form (one to two per day) or as capsules (two to four per day). Boldo is prepared as a tea (you can drink up to two cups [¹/₂ liter] a day), alone or mixed with other draining plants. In pharmacies and vitamin and health food stores, you'll find boldo teas in bags that will complete your hepatic (liver) detoxification. Headaches and digestive problems are signs that you've consumed too much; reduce the doses. Always remain progressive and patient.

▲ Kidney Detoxification

The kidneys also filter the blood, at the staggering rate of 4.2 cups (1 liter) per minute. We have two kidneys, located almost symmetrically on either side of our vertebral column at the bottom of the ribs (in the back of the body). These organs sort toxins and wastes to retain only what can no longer be reconverted. These last residues are evacuated directly through the urine, which is produced as needed, on average 1 milliliter per liter (or 0.2 teaspoon per 4.2 cups) of filtered blood. This production varies according to the quantity of toxins and wastes collected by the kidneys.

Urine production requires a basic liquid element, a sort of vital solvent—water. Contrary to what marketing slogans claim, water is more important for what it dissolves and drains out of the body than for what it brings to the body (mineral substances). If the kidneys don't receive enough water, the urine produced is more and more concentrated in wastes and this leads to a latent autointoxication of the renal (kidney) tissue itself. This is why the simplest way to detoxify the kidneys is to increase your consumption of water. But be careful: you must not overdo it and fatigue these delicate organs by an influx of liquid that is too large.

■ An adult man of average size (155 to 175 pounds) should drink between one liter and one-and-a-half liters of water per day, or six to eight medium-size glasses (6 to 7 ounces). The same applies for an adult woman of average size (120 to 135 pounds). Here again, this is an average, not the norm. Our needs for water vary according to the metabolism of each person and the quantity of wastes generated by day-to-day life. Highly stressed people, living in an environment heavy in atmospheric pollutions and consuming mostly industrialized foods, will produce more waste. Their body will need to receive more water in order to be able to eliminate those wastes. Some external elements also affect our needs for water: heat, intense physical activity, and the like must all be taken into account.

■ One essential rule of detoxification for everyone: Try to drink water at room temperature or barely cooled (never iced), taking small sips throughout the day. Stop drinking one half-hour before meals so as not to drown your alimentary bolus. During meals, don't drink more than one medium-size glass (6 to 7 ounces). Begin drinking again a half-hour after the end of the meal so as not to disturb digestion.

■ Choose noncarbonated water with few minerals that has a "high resistivity" and a "low coefficient of oxidation." These designations may seem a bit complicated or outlandish, but they're actually quite simple. They refer to the water's pH level, sodium level, and total dissolved solids level. To find out the quality of your tap water, contact your municipality's water services agency. For bottled water, carefully read the label and pick waters that have:

  ▪ a pH below 7.2
  ▪ a sodium level below 20 mg
  ▪ a dry residue at 180° lower than 350 mg per liter, which expresses the level of mineral salts in the water. This is the case for Évian, Volvic, and Vermont Pure waters, for example.

■ Avoid regularly consuming carbonated mineral waters with a lot of bicarbonate. Read the label carefully: the quantity of bicarbonates should not be higher than 700 mg per liter, because the kidneys must eliminate this surplus of minerals, and this unnecessarily fatigues them. Besides, the waters that are reputed to improve digestion have a tendency to impede it. Waters with digestive benefits are effective at the source, but they almost never are once they're bottled.

■ Avoid tap water, which has too much chlorine (a powerful cellular oxidant), or use a quality filtering system, either affixed to the faucet or in a carafe.

■ To improve this kidney detoxification, do a little treatment from time to time with draining herbal teas. Meadowsweet, orthosiphon, and mouse-ear hawkweed all gently activate the kidneys. Orthosiphon is usually taken as capsules or vials. Meadowsweet and mouse-ear hawkweed can be consumed together as a tea (10 grams of dried flowers for one bowl of boiling water; infuse for three minutes). Drink two mugs of the tea per day, with a little bit of honey, taking small sips.

▲ My Special Detox Formula for Cellular Problems

Thanks to my collaborations with excellent herbal doctors (working closely with medical teams at hospitals specializing in cancer treatment), I have found two detox formulas adapted for cancer patients that are effective and well tolerated by the body. I recommend them as herbal teas, not for the traditional aspect or the ecological benefit of these preparations, but for their deep biological effectiveness when compared with vials or capsules.

Horsetail

■ Measure 1 teaspoon dried horsetail for one large cup of boiling water, and infuse it for two minutes for the first three weeks of treatment, then three minutes during the weeks to follow. Drink two glasses per day (plain or with a bit of honey, if you prefer), one upon awakening and the other at around 6 p.m. Drink the tea warm, taking small sips (allocate half an hour to drink the entire cup).

A Felicitous Trio: Nettles, Yarrow, Marigold

■ Add daily to the horsetail the following dried herbs: 2 teaspoons marigold, 1 teaspoon yarrow, and 1 teaspoon nettles.

■ Add the above mix to one mug boiling water; let it infuse for two minutes. Drink two mugs per day (plain or with a bit of honey); one an hour and a half after breakfast, the other an hour and a half after lunch. Drink this tea, taking very small sips, very slowly (allow up to two hours to drink each cup). You can use a thermos to keep the tea warm.

These detox cures are well known in Germanic countries (Germany, Austria, Switzerland), where the phytotherapy tradition is alive and well. Herbal cleansings do not directly heal anything, but they figure in the overall care of your body and support of your healing processes.

▲ Other Herbal Detox Teas

Food plants (spices, herbs) are also true allies of detoxification. Here is a small selection of teas that will support the action of your organs of elimination without irritating your digestive tract, while exerting an alkalizing effect that will help neutralize the excess acidity of your internal environment. You can integrate these teas into your day as beverages to enjoy because they taste good.

■ Fennel: My favorite, and a fascinating plant. It acts on all the digestive functions. It supports the work of the liver and intestines in particular, and it's very alkalizing. Each morning for three weeks, prepare yourself a bottle of tea by infusing three tablespoons of fennel seeds in one liter of boiling water. It has a nice flavor and can be consumed plain or lightly sweetened with honey.

■ Green anise perfectly complements fennel, and the two can be mixed together. Its seeds have digestive benefits and notably stimulate the work of the gallbladder. The flavors of fennel and anise pair marvelously. Green anise tea is prepared with 2 tablespoons of seeds for 1 liter of boiling water. Infuse three minutes. Strain. If you wish to prepare a tea of fennel and anise combined, measure 2 tablespoons of fennel seeds and 1 tablespoon of anise seeds for 1 liter of boiling water, and let the tea infuse for three minutes. Strain.

■ Cumin seeds have an action similar to that of the other two: they are alkalizing, easily digested, and antitoxic. The recommended quantities to prepare a tea are 2 tablespoons for 1 liter of boiling water. Let it infuse for three minutes. Strain. Because its flavor is strong, you can lightly sweeten it by adding 1 tablespoon of honey for 1 liter of infusion (preferably thyme or rosemary honey, which both have detox virtues).

If you want to simplify the task, you'll find teas that are mixtures of these plants packaged in bags at better health food stores and co-ops.

DETOX NUTRITIONAL SUPPLEMENTS

Over the years reams of paper have been used to discuss pollution from heavy metals due largely to the increase in noxious gases in the atmosphere (lead from the fumes of motor vehicles and cadmium from secondhand cigarette smoke). Certain nutrients with antioxidants can effectively help us cleanse the body of heavy metals (the exact term is to *chelate*), while at the same time protecting our tissues from the excess production of free radicals (those famous accelerators of aging and cellular pollution).

As I've noted previously, I am very much in favor of taking antioxidants. But, again, better is the enemy of good enough. You must be careful to choose quality products from a reputable brand and not to exceed the recommended doses.

I generally suggest doing a three-week treatment (preferably with the change of seasons), choosing a nutritional supplement that has a balanced formula and physiological doses (the minimum dose needed to produce a physiological effect). Look for trusted brands with a good reputation, available at pharmacies and better health food and supplement stores.

Of course, if you've just been diagnosed with cancer, do not wait for the next change of season; rather, begin this treatment right away.

These anti–free radical and detox formulas* must at least contain vitamin C, vitamin E, selenium, magnesium, L-methionine, L-cystine, and bioflavonoids. Older formulas, containing only vitamins A, C, and E and selenium, are not well balanced. You must choose formulas without vitamins A, beta-carotene, vitamin B_6, and vitamin B_{12}, and combine them with magnesium in order to balance the two paths of production of free radicals in the mitochondria. If needed, take magnesium in the form of a trace element, in the amount of one capsule in the morning and one in the evening during the three weeks of the treatment.

FROM PERSONAL ECOLOGY
TO PLANETARY ECOLOGY

These practical considerations about our internal pollution lead me to a thought that constitutes the heart of my medical practice: each of us must realize that our body is our first planet (see appendix 1). Many of us think that the twenty-first century will be one of planetary ecology. We now see that grave ecological threats appear regularly, with pollution that implicates our long-term and even immediate survival. The pollution on our planet is a major challenge for this new century, for ourselves and especially for our children.

We are going to have to display a lot of clearheadedness, courage, and discipline if we are to resolve this worldwide problem. We need to develop these same qualities to resolve our own health problems. Ecology is an issue that is global, local, and individual. We will address it all the better once we have begun to take good care of our "planet body." Individually adopting a better "ecology of the body"—by refusing to pollute yourself daily with antihealth foods and beverages that have no nutritional value—is a first step toward better collectively addressing global issues.

I believe that this ecology of being (body, mind, and emotions)

---

*I do not specify doses because all the formulas are by recommended daily allowances (RDA) in accordance with the FDA to allow for correct, safe assimilation.

ought to precede an ecology of having (consumption, matter, planet). If we adopted an approach at the service of a more "human" being—one that focuses on moderating the consumption craze and its passion for accumulating material things—we could curb the pollution of our planet.

But, above all, I believe these Delta Detoxification tools will produce the beginnings of a metabolic smile from your polluted, exhausted organs.

Key Points

→ The production of multiple toxins and wastes is a normal consequence of cellular metabolism. These toxins must be eliminated regularly, just as the numerous pollutants coming from outside the body (nutritional, atmospheric) must be eradicated.

→ Our body has specialized organs for this, called *emunctories*. The most important of these are the liver, the kidneys, the intestines, the lungs, and the skin.

→ These organs are sometimes compromised, and this prevents them from doing their job well. At the same time, the quantity of wastes they must manage continues to increase.

→ When a body is affected by cancer (or a degenerative illness), the life scale is weighted toward the sick side. The least bit of additional weight on that side of the scale aggravates this imbalance.

→ All cancers call for intense, toxic chemical treatments, which demand additional effort from the organs of elimination.

→ The Delta Detoxification treatments do not directly heal the body. But they help to lighten the workload and facilitate the functioning of the organs of elimination, which allows the body to more easily mobilize all its healing forces.

→ To facilitate intestinal detoxification, you must emphasize hydration and regular bowel movements; prunes and fiber supplements are valuable aids.

→ To facilitate liver detoxification, you can consume black radish (in vials), artichoke (in vial or capsule form), and boldo (as a tea).

→ To facilitate kidney detoxification, you must drink enough water (a water low in minerals, at room temperature, sipped throughout the day), as well as herbal teas: meadowsweet, orthosiphon, or mouse-ear hawkweed.

→ If you're diagnosed with cancer, you must consume my two detox teas: (1) horsetail tea, and (2) a mixture of nettles, yarrow, and marigold.

→ During your convalescence from cancer treatment, to give overall support to the detoxification forces of the body, you must drink infusions of fennel seed, cumin, and green anise.

→ There are also excellent nutritional supplements in the form of plants and antioxidants that promote detoxification. Quality and safety are of the utmost importance. Ask your doctor or nutritionist for advice. Read labels carefully; certain micronutrients are to be avoided in cases of cellular problems, including vitamin A, beta-carotene, vitamin B_6, and vitamin B_{12}.

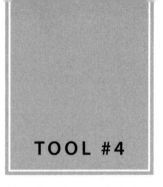

TOOL #4

DELTA RELAXATION

It's a deceptively simple enemy that can in large part be blamed for diseases of civilization: stress.
DENNIS T. JAFFE, *HEALING FROM WITHIN*

Excess stress is the certified enemy of our health and healing process. Once this stress is revealed, all that needs to be done to heal is to fight it effectively.

But as Edmund Jacobson, widely considered the originator of modern relaxation techniques, explains, "The individual usually doesn't know which muscles are tense, cannot accurately judge if he is relaxed, and doesn't clearly realize what he must do to relax. Moreover, he doesn't know how to do it. These abilities must be learned, or rediscovered." Jacobson created a famous method of systematic relaxation called Jacobson Progressive Relaxation.

Delta Relaxation, the fourth tool for health, will help you rediscover or learn the best antistress techniques.

Up to now, the tools of Delta Medicine that I have outlined have been centered on the direct improvement of your physiological functioning. You have learned how to breathe better, eat better, and cleanse your body of excess waste and internal and external pollution. We will now head to the more subtle territory of neurobiology and physiology to follow paths less frequented but no less effective. We are going to enter the mind-body domain.

As explained in previous chapters, mind-body medicine deals with medical techniques that are rooted in simple psychological training (such as mental imagery, or MI) that results in real modifications to our biological equilibrium. Mind-body practice deals with other types of techniques based on gentle physical training that prompts modifications in our psychological and nervous equilibrium.

Together, these two complementary fields of action demonstrate to what degree our body, through all the complexity of its biological and metabolic manifestations, is closely connected to our mind (see scientific references for this in appendix 3). A direct therapeutic application results from it: by acting on one or the other of these elements (the body in one case, thoughts in the other), each day we can introduce small positive impacts (Delta impulses) that will weigh heavier and heavier on the healthy side of our life balance, thus neutralizing the impact of unhealthy thoughts and negative pressures and allowing us to flourish. This is what Delta Relaxation offers by way of simple health techniques to put into practice on a daily basis.

STRESS, IMMUNITY, AND THE ENDOCRINE SYSTEM

Our autonomic, or involuntary, nervous system (with its two branches—sympathetic and parasympathetic) is located at the juncture of the mind-body connection. It relays the impacts of stress, nervous tension, and emotional shocks within our body. These repeated impacts end up weakening and destabilizing our nervous system, which we now know is connected to both the endocrine and immune systems.

Here is one example among hundreds, often observed (and too often neglected): thousands of women will confirm that during times when they have undergone intense emotional pressure or ongoing stress, they experienced hormonal disorders that disrupted their menstrual cycle (sometimes to the point of stopping their period altogether), altered their fertility (sterility of a psychological origin), or caused a miscarriage. The effects of stress can also manifest themselves at menopause, which progresses more smoothly when the woman is not under stress on a psychological or emotional level. By learning to better manage stress and emotions, we can soften these life impacts and preserve the harmony of the neurohormonal system. Such impacts also play a role in the creation of millions of gastric ulcers each year (associated with the bacteria *Helicobacter pylori* and too much stress) and the thousands of sadly commonplace heart attacks.

Excess nervous tension and emotional shocks (abrupt or repeated over time) also have an impact on the functioning of the immune system (this is the domain of psychoneuroimmunology.) You have probably noticed recurring fever blisters (herpes) on yourself or someone close to you. Like colds, they often appear at the end of a vacation, or on Monday morning when it's time to return to work. These pathological manifestations are not far-fetched imaginings. They're due to the temporary lowering of immunity that follows stress: in the case above, the prospect of diving back into a professional activity that is perceived as particularly burdensome or stressful.

Many studies have explored the relationship between stress and emotions on the one hand, and immunity on the other. A team of researchers in Boston, for example, followed a group of students at a dental school during one entire school year. They regularly took saliva samples to measure the students' immunoglobulin levels. (Immunoglobulins are central to the defense reactions of the body, notably in helping to create antibodies.) This level remained nearly stable throughout the year but fell when exams approached. The decrease was especially significant among anxious students and those whose parents were worried about their children's academic achievement (pressure to succeed).

Studies were carried out on animals, also sensitive to stress. One team of researchers studied two groups of identical rats from the same litter. They were fed the same way and lived in the same environment. But the animals in one of the groups received small electric shocks from time to time (randomly). These shocks were not painful but made their life uncomfortable. For three weeks the growth of the animals remained identical between the two groups (same weight, same size). But after twenty-five days, their biological constants began to vary considerably: the rats subjected to the uncomfortable situation saw their immune defenses crumble. They had crossed over their Delta Point of resistance to stress.

Scientists no longer have any doubts on the subject: stress, nervous tension, and negative emotions have observable and measurable repercussions on our vitality and the state of our health. These psychosomatic repercussions affect us in dozens of ways, but the specifics of their physiological progression and biological equations are not yet fully understood. The same quality of stress won't produce the same illness or the same symptoms in two different people (because their biological and nervous terrains are different). This complicates a purely symptomatic approach. It's no longer just about treating an organ or a sick system, but now we must address the person's body, mind, and overall personality. The investment in therapeutic time and human time is necessarily much more important. This, no doubt, explains the "polite marginalization" of all types of mind-body therapy, even if they're medically recognized as being useful and effective. These techniques nevertheless constitute the preferred sphere for healing. They are often very effective and, for the most part, easy to learn, practice, and apply.

Delta Relaxation fits easily within the context of mind-body medicine, so rich in influences on our healing and health. Using certain kinds of phrases, repeated silently while in a state of relaxation and with the objective of healing, we can see a balancing and harmonizing effect on our entire nervous system. And this calming message resonates out to the other vital functions, notably the hormonal and immune systems. The nervous, hormone, and immune systems are all strongly implicated in cases of cancer.

THE MIND-BODY CONNECTION

"The separation of psychology from the premises of biology is purely artificial, because the human psyche lives in indissoluble union with the body." Spoken intuitively by the great Carl Gustav Jung, the scientific reality of mind-body medicine took a century to develop and is now solidly established as a reference point for all the neurosciences.

It all began with the Nobel Prize in 1904, crowning the work of the famous Ivan Pavlov. His studies proved the theory of conditioned reflexes: by associating a dog's meal with the sound of a bell, after several weeks the dog's digestive system started to function upon hearing the ring of the bell, without eating any food. This major discovery confirmed for the first time dozens of observations and clarified medical symptoms that were until then mysterious: some people who were allergic to plants or animals would suffer from a serious allergic reaction at the mere sight of a photograph of the allergen (and without the presence of it). This demonstrated the existence of a bridge between the mind, the hormonal system, and the immune system. But the biological schema of this bridge would remain a mystery for more than half a century.

It wasn't until the 1970s that Nicolas Cohen and Robert Ader presented an even more precise psychobiological schema: rats were fed concentrated sugar water mixed with a toxic immune suppressant, causing death within weeks of regular administration. But if during the experiment the toxic medicine was removed from the sugar water, the rat still died, even in the absence of the mortal dose. It was as if the immune system of the rat believed that it was still drinking poison while only drinking sugar water.

The connection between the nervous and immune systems was proved. Several years later David Felten finally demonstrated that nervous connections (the mysterious bridges) were directly connected to lymphoid tissue (the immune system). The nervous system was therefore this physiological bridge between the mind (thoughts) and the immune system (certain cells of the body). It was Ader who came up with the term *psychoneuroimmunology* for this new scientific field that would guide the birth of neuroscience.

With these new bases of overall comprehension, everything became clearer and, above all, more coherent. An excess of accumulated nervous tension provokes physical and mental chronic fatigue, and this sets the stage for numerous degenerative pathologies, called lifestyle diseases, or diseases of civilization. This deleterious action has repercussions on several levels, like a morbid cascade. It first leads to a targeted organic weakening (adrenal glands, then thymus). This, in turn, causes a suppression of immune activity (overall or targeted), which can cause the appearance of a number of disorders, such as autoimmune or certain degenerative diseases.

Beyond these direct consequences, mental and nervous fatigue bring about a decrease in daily lucidity in the short term, and therefore impair the control we exert over the course of our lives. The resulting mood changes can rapidly turn into depression that may become clinical.

All the techniques of Delta Relaxation are rooted in these findings. From the end of the nineteenth century up until the mid-twentieth century, some of these techniques (notably suggestion and medical hypnosis) had been identified and used in clinics and hospitals.* They are not mysterious, marginal, or "alternative." They play an integral part in the history and success of modern medicine (Sainte-Anne Hospital in Paris is an international point of reference for the quality and originality of its treatments; see appendix 3).

In fact, all you need to do is refer to the etymological meaning of the term *psychosomatic* to grasp its general sense and the implications. It joins the Greek roots *psyche* and *soma,* the first designating the overall

---

*Medical hypnosis was studied by Jean-Martin Charcot at the Pitié-Salpêtrière Hospital in Paris in the 1880s. The experiments he conducted were mostly on people suffering from hysteria and epilepsy. The young Freud studied hypnosis with Charcot before turning to the "talking cure," later called *psychoanalysis.* See appendix 3.

group of mental phenomena, the second those of the body. This combination creates a linguistic bridge between these two universes: *psychosomatic* refers to all approaches that unite, in a cause-and-effect relationship, mental actions (and manifestations) and their physical (or somatic) consequences. More simply, this term, as a medical therapeutic tool, designates the influence of our thoughts (as words or images) on our body.

Everyone has experienced psychosomatic phenomena, most often, unfortunately, in a negative way. We know that an excess of stress can disturb digestion and cause disagreeable burning sensations in the stomach. If not properly treated, this can lead to a latent inflammatory state that results in ulcers. And if the patient does not receive prompt medical attention—in order to identify the initial stress and modify the patient's biological terrain—the ulcer may even morph into cancer. This same pattern characterizes the onset of all sorts of pathologies, from allergies to insomnia, and includes cutaneous disorders (eczema, psoriasis), gynecological disorders, chronic fatigue, and chronic depression.

Therefore, thoughts that aren't well controlled or directed, as well as unmanaged stress, can be enough to provoke biological and psychological disturbances that are very real. And if people under stress don't succeed in regaining inner calm and serenity, they can slowly slide from mental upset into a true symptomatic illness. This illness will no longer have any direct connection with the thoughts that engendered it, but that does not lessen the consequences. Keep in mind that psychosomatic illnesses are just as real as others; they are not at all imaginary. But their causes are more difficult to pinpoint, and their classification is not as well codified in Western medicine.

I have given some extreme examples. But this type of psychopathological process can also take place without reaching such bitter ends. Don't certain thoughts lead us to blush or turn pale? Others make our heart beat faster or cause us to gasp. We've all experienced these reactions and have integrated them into our daily lives. They are nonetheless very good examples of purely psychosomatic reactions, of psycho-organic biological patterns.

From these universal observations it is easy to imagine a form of "therapeutic reciprocity": thoughts that are better controlled and better directed will cause physical reactions that are no longer negative but instead positive, moving in the direction of well-being, healing, and health. All the tools of Delta Relaxation are based on the major scientific findings of Ivan Pavlov, Alfred Adler, and David Felten. Our mental training uses these therapeutic connections, intertwined to influence, support, and reinforce the processes of healing. Taking a serious interest in the field in the 1980s, several universities (American, Canadian, and French) opened their own departments of psychoneuroimmunology.

MIND-BODY INTERACTION

The path of mind-body medicine can lead in both directions. We've all experienced the processes of psychoemotional calming in response to relaxation or bodily well-being. This is what happens when you dive into a hot bath after a stressful, exhausting day. By relieving your body of some of its weight, the water removes the task of constantly managing and adapting to earth's gravity, freeing the brain. This first reaction, originating in the body, spreads to the neurocerebral realm by inducing relaxation—first nervous, then mental. The warmth of the water contributes to the process. Added to this, no doubt, is an echo produced deep within the layers of your psyche that awakens sensations imprinted during your intrauterine existence, when you were cradled by maternal movements, protected in the warmth of the amniotic liquid. The result: Within ten minutes you feel your nervous tension dissipating, and a mental calming takes over.

While seemingly banal, this example clearly shows the way in which gestures, actions, and physical contexts can have repercussions on our psyche. As with psychosomatic illness, these intimately linked processes can act in both directions. All of us have felt a sense of insidious depression worm its way inside us and mix up our emotions when we feel physically fatigued. Luckily, it is possible to induce relaxation and bodily harmony that will help fight nervous fatigue. This is the other branch of Delta Relaxation.

ILLNESS ANNOUNCED: A MAJOR SOURCE OF STRESS

Let's return for a moment to the place where we started: we were all born in good health (except, of course, those born with genetic pathologies), and each one of our cells possesses this memory; each one of our cells retains the memory and the imprint of this point of reference and of the forces of healing. Certain gestures, certain attitudes, certain thoughts, and certain mistakes made in daily life have contributed to the construction of the illness in our body; but (and this is fundamental) other gestures, other attitudes, other thoughts can help reverse this process and deconstruct the forces that are disturbing our innermost equilibrium. All the tools of Delta Medicine are therefore aimed at awakening our memory of health and mobilizing all our healing forces.

Nevertheless, the patients that I've treated are unanimous on one point: when they heard for the first time the words *serious disease* from a doctor, they felt very uneasy, and some were nauseated or dizzy, as if they were about to pass out. Vomiting or fainting: one corresponds to an attempt to reject the terrible news, the other to a wish to flee from the intolerable.*

It's very difficult to accept the diagnosis of a serious disease, because no one is prepared for it. The news calls up deep-rooted fears and worries. Yet we all consciously know that our life could be interrupted at any moment: all it would take is a second of inattention at the steering

---

*This observation concerns about 90 percent of people diagnosed with serious illness. There are also paradoxical reactions (joy, laughter, amusement, serenity) in which neurotic nervous compensations arise, as well as true latent processes of bravery and a determination to combat the illness and triumph over it. This is all to be taken into account within the dialogue space that each therapist must offer the patient.

wheel or while crossing the street for our life to change radically. Of course, we don't think about that every day (it would be too depressing). Besides, our unconscious (which is trained to write our emotions and memories) perceives itself as immortal. As a result, in a more or less stable state of equilibrium between the conscious and the unconscious, none of us is ever ready to hear that our life is in danger. None of us will calmly welcome the reminder of our mortal condition.

When we are given the diagnosis of a serious disease, our sense of our own omnipotence is shaken. We are brutally brought back to the unacceptable fragility of our life and our daily equilibrium. A sick person desperately tries to reject or flee all this the moment when disease is announced.

The Delta Relaxation exercises—combined with the Delta Breathing exercises—are particularly (and immediately) useful in helping you get through the toughest step: standing up to oppressive, negative thoughts brought on by the announcement of the disease, and then substituting constructive thoughts that will prompt you to mobilize all those invaluable healing forces.

CALMING AND RECONCILIATION

Let's pay close attention to the next step: you now wear the label of *sick person*. The medical team has assigned this somewhat brutal diagnosis to you, and it makes you uneasy, generating wide-ranging fears and anxieties. A mass of cells has been built inside your body. You don't have control over it, and the doctors call it a *tumor*, or a blood cancer, like leukemia. No matter what the case, if you consciously accept the fact that this illness "belongs" to you, you will have a much easier time helping your body deconstruct it.

From the moment the diagnosis is made, the first work must then be one of calming and acceptance in the form of Delta Breathing exercises, combined with specific thoughts. This stage of positive acceptance (rather than capitulation) is very important when it comes to the progress of the disease. This specific disease (this one, and no other) has developed in this specific body (yours, with its strengths and weaknesses). It is "your" disease. If you reject it and hate it, you reject and hate yourself at the same time. The more you try to deny it, the more you will drain yourself of the energy you need to fight it, or, more precisely, to understand it better and deconstruct it.

Don't forget that the imbalances that have accumulated over the years express themselves through your most fragile organ, the one whose weakness is inscribed in your genetic life book. Imagine a dozen people storming a mountain's summit. Those who are exhausted first will always be those in the worst shape—the ones to easily tire, the weakest physically and psychologically. As the climbers' ascent continues, exhaustion comes to the others little by little; among those who are left, the least resistant succumb next. In the end, only the strongest remain.

It's the same with our tissues, organs, and cells. The weakest are the first affected by illness. By any logic, we should want to help them, support them, save them. Not only because they are the most fragile but also because they have made themselves the brave and generous messengers of our imbalances. They tell us, translate for us, some of our erroneous behaviors. They also point out some of our faults. Sometimes they even cry out to us that we are not maintaining the good health we had when we came into the world. But most often we reject the afflicted area, along with the illness that we want to get rid of radically, like amputating a gangrenous limb or trying to cut out a cancerous organ with surgery.

Are the liver, prostate, ovaries, or lungs affected by disease? We sometimes turn our attention away from these organs, as if they were responsible for the disaster that has befallen us. We somehow feel betrayed by the sick organ. We might even hate it. We might want to tell it, "Why are you doing this to me? We're part of the same body!" These reactions are tainted with negative emotions (a sense of injustice, anger) that may disturb our nervous, metabolic, and immune equilibrium even further.

Instead of repeating these reproaches, we should send the organ messages of support. It's an ally, a friend all the more devoted for accepting to suffer (to be sick) in order to reveal to us our life imbalances.

Some of the Delta Relaxation exercises are specifically created to help you establish this indispensable reconciliation within yourself. All you need to do is begin a form of symbolic benevolent dialogue with your organs while in a state of relaxation, with the help of selected words and mental imagery that will become therapeutic. The power of mind-body medicine will do the rest.

FOR THOSE UNDERGOING RADIATION THERAPY OR CHEMOTHERAPY

In almost all types of cancer, patients are obligated to undergo aggressive treatments—chemotherapy or radiation therapy. They generally know that these treatments are effective but also toxic to the organs and the body's healthy tissues. Therefore, some people harbor a very negative image of the treatment and go to the treatment sessions reluctantly. During the sessions they try to distract themselves any way they can to forget about the brutality their body is suffering in an attempt to return to health.

In my experience this approach produces the same negative effects as denying the illness or rejecting the sick organ. When these treatments are prescribed, they are essential to your treatment protocol. They can truly give you access to healing. The procedure has been established by specialists, doctors with enough experience and expertise to select the treatments best suited to remedy your condition.

But to get the most out of these treatments it is crucial to understand them (by having them clearly explained) and then accept them. If you make the effort to concentrate during the chemo or radiation session, conscious of the battle taking place inside your body, you will optimize the effectiveness of the treatment. You will mobilize your confidence about its benefits rather than exacerbating your fears about the possible negative side effects. (Remember: chemotherapy is a valuable tool for healing. Focusing on this thought will support your body in its fight against the cancer.) I offer a very specific way to do this (see page 154), one that my patients always practice with satisfying results, both mentally and physically.

Let me make clear that in no way do I claim that Delta Relaxation makes chemotherapy more effective, nor that it directly diminishes its side effects. (However, the indirect positive influence—a progressive, directed mobilization of the body's blood flow—has now been scientifically proved and is better and better understood biologically.) Delta Relaxation does allow you to better manage the neuropsychological (and sometimes physical) impact of these aggressive treatments. The exercise helps to awaken our mind-body healing forces that, while very different from one person to the next, always triumph over illness when stimulated and always compromise our immune system when weakened.

Many people have been pleasantly surprised by practicing these Delta Relaxation exercises during their chemo or radiation sessions, but I can't guarantee that this will be the case for you. On the other hand, I can assure you of one thing: instead of arriving at the treatments full of anxiety and stress, you'll learn to approach them with serenity. And the repercussions of this mental state are always beneficial to the prognosis.

DELTA RELAXATION:
THE JUNCTURE OF MIND-BODY MEDICINE

Delta Relaxation will thus ameliorate all situations inherent in an illness, from the announcement of the diagnosis up to and through the treatments themselves. These tools for health lie at the juncture of mind-body interaction. They act on the mind to calm the body, and they act on the body to calm the mind.

Many techniques exist in this domain: medical hypnosis, sophrology, Jacobson's progressive muscle relaxation, and, above all, the autogenic therapy of Dr. Johannes Heinrich Schultz, who inspired a century of therapists. Schultz was a doctor, a neurologist, and a psychiatrist. At the end of the nineteenth century he was one of the first doctors to take an interest in the close relationship between the body and the mind. He studied our natural capacities for self-hypnosis and self-persuasion and succeeded in standardizing them so that we can put ourselves in a beneficial state of relaxation at any moment.

The Delta Relaxation exercises that I offer here use the most practical methods of autogenous training, combined with breathing exercises and directed work on thoughts that have been standardized and refined from year to year. All this now gives you a unique tool for health aimed at the healing process. Mental imagery is an important element of numerous mind-body techniques. Dr. Schultz used it frequently with his students to point out to them the relationship between thoughts and the body. For example, he knew how to direct and intensify at will the blood flow to different parts of his body. Sometimes at the beginning of one of his classes he would take off his shirt, lie on his back, and announce to his students that his throat hurt too much to talk. To heal the sore throat, he would relax and imagine that his blood flowed to this painful area, bringing with it all the naturally calming substances that the body can produce. Within minutes the students, astounded, observed that his throat and the top of his shoulders were turning bright red and hot, proof that the blood flow had "obeyed" his silent command. He was able to work in the same way with his hands, his feet, his forehead, and his face.

To understand this stunning mind-body exercise, here is a little practical experiment that you can do right now. It will only take you two or three minutes.

- Sit down or lie down in a comfortable position and close your eyes. Breathe deeply and relax.
- Now imagine that you are holding a nice ripe lemon in your hands. In your mind, touch its yellow skin, still warm from the sun's rays. Smell its scent.

• Continue these sensations for a minute or two. Then imagine that you cut the lemon in two and hold one half up to your mouth. Now take a great, big bite into the sour flesh.

The moment when you imagined biting into the lemon, odds are you felt your salivary glands contract slightly and an influx of saliva invaded your mouth. The idea of the lemon, its mental image associated with the sour flavor, made you (in reality) salivate that way.

In the same way, you can influence the functioning of your nervous system with controlled thoughts and guided mental imagery. This domain of neuroscience is called MI (mental imagery). You can't totally master the ortho- and parasympathetic systems by force of thoughts and mental imagery alone, because they function, above all, in an unconscious way. But these images influence the mental control that guides these systems by promoting better nervous equilibrium and greater resistance to nervous and emotional tensions. Or, put more simply, better mind-body harmony guarantees greater vitality of our healing mechanisms.

DELTA RELAXATION IN PRACTICE

We will start with a mind-body relaxation, followed by an exercise centered on the dynamic acceptance of the disease. Then I'll suggest that you create within yourself a state of calm and serenity (which you can "lean on" for nervous and moral support). You'll then be able to learn to relax your body and your mind, thanks to these simple physical exercises. Finally, I will suggest an exercise that is essential to practice if you are undergoing chemotherapy or radiation therapy.

▲ "I Visualize My Body Relaxed"

■ Lie down in a quiet place or, if that isn't possible, sit down in a comfortable position or settle into the coachman's position (see page 59). Relax, release the muscles of your body, and close your eyes.

- Breathe deeply three times (always through the nose), then adopt a regular breathing rhythm without forcing the breath. Breathe in, counting to three (one one thousand, two one thousand, three one thousand), then breathe out slowly, counting to six (one one thousand, two one thousand, three one thousand, four one thousand . . .). Repeat three times.

- Now bring your attention to your feet (a part of the body often forgotten). Imagine they are relaxed, that all the muscles release and they become heavier and heavier (as if they were gently sinking into the ground).

- Still breathing calmly and without effort, draw your "inner gaze" up to your ankles, your legs, your knees, your thighs, your pelvis, then up to your stomach and to your ribs. Once they are relaxed, feel the "weight" in each of these parts of the body.

- You've arrived at the shoulders. Give this area of the body a little more attention until it is very relaxed; it's often the object of multiple tensions (we carry the weight of the world on our shoulders).

- Now descend along the arms to the elbows, the forearms, the wrists, and the hands (relaxed, becoming heavier and heavier).

- Finally, relax your face and your forehead. Slightly part your lips to form the hint of a smile, your breath calm and regular.

- Feel your body becoming heavy, as if it were sinking into the chair or mattress. Enjoy this sensation for a few moments. Then follow the same path through your body, this time in the other direction—from your head to your toes.

- Slowly repeat this deep relaxation and progressive "weightiness" of the body, up and then down, three times.

- Finally, bring your attention back to your breathing rhythm for a minute before opening your eyes, keeping a small smile (without forcing it).

If you practice this visualization regularly, you will soon notice that it creates an overall physical relaxation of the major muscle groups. It's a first, indispensable step on the path to mind-body relaxation and health. One fundamental point that applies to all the Delta Relaxation exercises: The more you practice, the more quickly the feeling of relaxation will come, and the more long-lasting the feeling of well-being will be.

▲ "I Make Peace with the Sick Organ"

- Lie down in a quiet place, or if this isn't possible, sit down in a comfortable position or settle in to the coachman's position. Relax, release the muscles of your body, and close your eyes.
- Breathe deeply three times (always through the nose), then adopt a regular breathing rhythm without forcing the breath. Breathe in, counting to three (one one thousand, two one thousand, three one thousand), then breathe out slowly, counting to six (one one thousand, two one thousand, three one thousand, four one thousand . . .). Repeat three times.
- Now imagine (visualize) your sick organ. You can choose how you'll form this representation: look at an image or a photograph of the organ in a dictionary or an anatomy book or online to inspire you, or let your imagination create a more or less schematic or fanciful representation. What's most important is that the image speaks to you.
- Next, send a wave of serenity to this sick organ. The most commonly used image is a beautiful white or gold light, calming and beneficial, that bathes the sick organ.
- Anchor this image with an accompanying statement. Repeat it silently to the organ: "I'm aware that you are suffering for me, and I thank you." And "Now I send you the strength of this light to help you and to heal you." When you pronounce these words, it's as if you have sent both gratitude and new healing forces to your body (the two mix in the overall positive effects of mind-body practice).
- Repeat each step of this visualization seven times. Then concentrate again on your breathing rhythm as you slowly return to normal consciousness. Then open your eyes.

Remember, if you aren't accustomed to therapeutic training, don't let your mind judge or criticize you: "What you're doing is stupid," "This is a waste of time," "These are just childish words," "Words don't heal," etc. Keep in mind that anything big that is done in the world always occurs by way of bravery and words. Calmly persevere for at least ten days: this is how long it takes to tame the critical thoughts coming from your fearful unconscious.

▲ "I Create Calm within Me"

- Lie down in a quiet place, or if this isn't possible, sit down in a comfortable position or settle in to the coachman's position. Relax, release the muscles of your body, and close your eyes.
- Breathe deeply three times (always through the nose), then adopt a regular breathing rhythm without forcing the breath. Breathe in, counting to three (one one thousand, two one thousand, three one thousand), then breathe out slowly, counting to six (one one thousand, two one thousand, three one thousand, four one thousand . . .). Repeat three times.
- Then as you inhale, stop counting and repeat to yourself one time: "I inhale and I know that I inhale." As you exhale, repeat to yourself twice: "I exhale and I know that I exhale." Repeat three times.
- Next, repeat to yourself as you inhale: "I inhale and I am calmer," and as you exhale: "I exhale and I am calmer." Repeat three times.
- Over the course of these relaxation sessions, you can vary the content of the statements: "I inhale energy for my body and I exhale to give this energy to my body," or "I inhale serenity and I exhale to release all tension."
- Practical remark: Either you see this beneficial energy (or light) in your body become luminous or full of healing energy, or you see a brown, gray, or black substance chase away the illness that you send
- Repeat each step of this relaxation three times, then bring your attention back to the breathing rhythm before opening your eyes.

▲ "I Relax a Key Area of My Body"

- This exercise is practiced standing (see page 61).
- Begin with the breathing exercises and head movements explained on pages 62–69.

- Then lift your shoulders while drawing in your head (as if you were going to hide it between your shoulders; see figure 1). Next, lift your head as you lower your shoulders (as if you were touching the sky with the top of your head; see figure 2). Do this movement three times.
- Now roll your shoulders three times back, then forward three times (see figure 3).

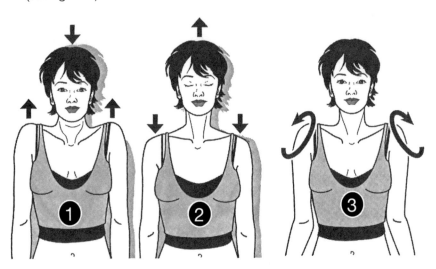

- Stand with your legs shoulder width apart, bend your knees slightly, and tilt your pelvis slightly forward as if you were trying to press it against the wall in front of you (see figure 4).
- In this posture, inhale as you lift your arms to the side so that they're parallel with the ground (see figure 5, movement A). Let your hands drop and turn the palms of your hands toward your forearm. Then lower your arms as you exhale, lifting your hands in the other direction so that the palms of your hands point to the ground (see figure 5, movement B). Your back and head remain straight but without any tension.
- Do this seven times.
- Finally, balance on one foot and then the other for a few seconds by slightly lifting each leg to the side for the same amount of time (see figure 6).
- Do this exercise seven times.

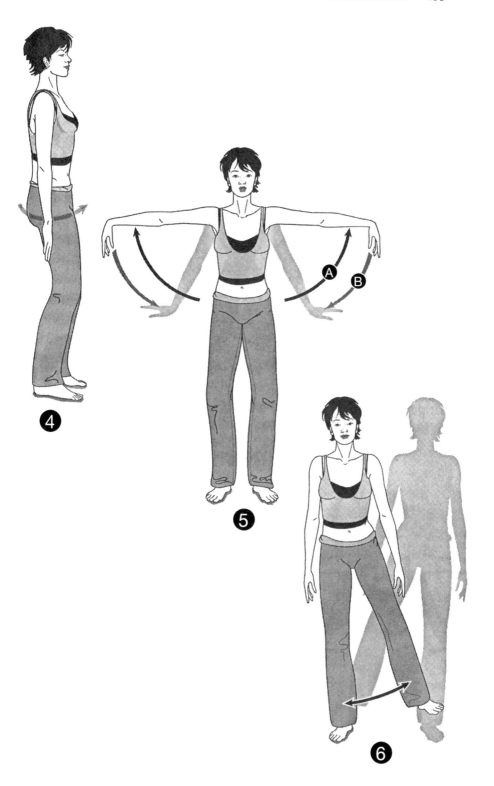

▲ Exercise to Accompany Chemotherapy or Radiation Therapy

I encourage patients who must undergo chemotherapy or radiation therapy to first follow the Delta Relaxation (beginning on page 134) and the Delta Detoxification (beginning on page 118) regimens for ten to fifteen days before the treatments begin. This will prepare their body to receive and metabolize the chemical molecules or therapeutic rays.

Then I urge them to do the following exercise each day during the entire duration of the treatment. In my experience, it is a key tool.

- In the morning upon wakening, do the basic breathing exercises for five to ten minutes to prepare your body for what it will take on during the day: concentrate on your breath and emphasize the exhalation, making it twice as long as the inhalation (see page 64).
- When you are settling in to receive the IV or the therapeutic rays, do the basic breathing exercise again and maintain this breathing pattern throughout the entire session.
- If this is a chemotherapy session, look calmly at the bag (or bottle) of liquid from which the IV flows, then close your eyes and imagine that it is not toxic to your body, but rather that it is beneficial. (In reality, as aggressive and toxic as these products may be, they are essentially—and primarily—therapeutic.)
- While retaining the rhythm and amplitude of your breathing, imagine that the chemo bag is filled with a luminous liquid that is white, yellow, or gold. Associate it with a feeling of power and confidence.
- As you inhale, see the luminous liquid flow out of the bag, travel through the tubes, and enter your veins to arrive at your heart, which welcomes it. Then, as you exhale, see this healing liquid, propelled by your heart, continue its path inside your body to the sick organ. See this luminous liquid spread into the smallest vessels of your body and flood them with its healing force, making your circulatory system entirely luminous.
- If you must undergo a radiation session, proceed in the same way and

visualize the invisible rays diffused by the machine in the form of golden light, and then imagine them penetrating your body to heal the sick organ.

■ These dynamic images must be combined with a sense of serenity, confidence, and inner peace. If, at the beginning, you still feel worried, you should know that the more you positively program your mind, the more a space of peace will grow within you, leaving less and less room for your fears.

These aren't simple mental images that I'm putting at the service of your healing. These are chosen images and directed thoughts, acting on a prepared emotional terrain. This type of mental imagery has nothing to do with magic. On their own, these images cannot direct the molecules of the medicine or the therapeutic rays solely to the sick area. But this exercise allows patients to participate fully in their treatment, and this promotes mobilization of the healing forces. With regular training, you will be able to influence your blood flow, as Dr. Schultz did. These directed visualizations will place you at the heart of your battle with the illness. You'll become your body's partner and help it face the situation head-on. The joint forces of healing (medicine) and self-healing (programmed mental imagery) will generate maximum healing, creating within you (and for you) new life energies.

Sometimes several patients are together in the same room while they receive chemotherapy, and they will share their impressions during the session, watch television, or listen to music. Some of my patients have admitted that when this happens they sometimes feel embarrassed to practice visualization in the company of other people who are taking a chemotherapy session at the same time, because the exercise cuts off the possibility of communication and conviviality. I suggest that they speak openly about it to the others and explain what they are doing in all seriousness and without embarrassment.

More than once I've received reports that the idea spread, and within a few sessions everyone was practicing the same exercise at the same time with a sense of conviviality that was silent but joyful and confident.

I'll add that this technique is totally respectful of the people treating you: it doesn't bother them at all; it is perfectly credible and discreet. Furthermore, it provides a sense of serenity rapidly apparent to other people nearby, who then feel the beneficial effects themselves. Many patients have told me that upon leaving the chemotherapy sessions in which they practiced this visualization, they didn't feel troubled, worried, or uncomfortable. They were calm and at ease. This is explained by the fact that they had practiced both the Delta Breathing and the Delta Relaxation for long enough that it calmed their nervous system; the images added even more to the positive mind-body force of the exercise. As the adage goes, a good example is the best teacher, so everyone wanted to know their secret. A very simple secret, and two little tools for health transformed into dynamic partners for healing.

Key Points

→ Our mind and body are closely connected, in health and in illness. The sum of stress and nervous tension weighs very heavily on the sick side of our life balance, contributing to the appearance of many forms of cellular problems.

→ By acting on one of these (mind or body), we can obtain effects on the other. This is the guiding principle of mind-body medicine. Each helps balance and regulate the other.

→ The nervous system sends the effects of stress and emotional shocks through the body. Because the nervous system undergoes repeated pressures from this stress and these emotional shocks, it ends up growing weaker, and this leads to reactions in the immune and hormonal systems, which are closely connected to the nervous system.

→ Many scientific studies have arrived at the same conclusion: the negative impact of all our nervous tension weakens the defenses of our immune system and our hormonal balance, as well as numerous other vital systems (digestion, sleep) that are key to our health.

→ Physical disorders can have a significant impact on our mental state. Chronic pain, for example, can cause depression.

→ When a person is affected by a serious disease, the negative impact from the stress of that illness is often intense. That compounds the numerous imbalances that have contributed to the construction of the illness within the body.

→ Delta Relaxation allows us to diminish the negative impact of stress and minimize the stress generated by the announcement and the context of the disease.

→ Delta Relaxation incorporates calming work and reconciliation with the organ or function affected by the illness.

→ The Delta Relaxation exercises combine breath training, visualization, and directed work on reprogramming thoughts.

→ Special body training that borrows techniques from mind-body medicine helps the body to relax deeply, calming nervous tension and anxious thoughts.

→ A specific exercise of directed visualization, practiced during radiation therapy and chemotherapy sessions, helps patients deal with the stress generated by these treatments and potentially limits the negative side effects of these treatments.

→ With your newfound serenity you'll serve as an example to those in distress around you and will be able to help them, too.

→ Be aware that recommending a good book or a competent therapist is well meaning. However, taking on the burden of another's emotional upset is something else altogether. Avoid this trap at all costs, even if you feel compelled to step in. Generously share reference books and practical guides, but save all your new "nervous energy" for yourself until you are fully healed.

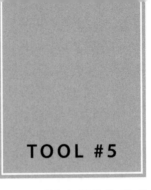

TOOL #5

DELTA PSYCHOLOGY

The human mind is a great lever, and the treating doctor must use this lever.

HIPPOLYTE BERNHEIM

"All I mean is that we shouldn't behave like rabbits and put our complete trust in doctors. For instance, I'm reading this book." He picked up a large, open book from the windowsill. "Abrikosov and Stryukov, *Pathological Anatomy*, medical school textbook. It says here that the link between the development of tumors and the central nervous system has so far been very little studied. And this link is an amazing thing! It's written here in so many words." He found the place. "'It happens rarely, but there are cases of self-induced healing.' You see how it's worded? Not recovery through treatment, but actual healing." . . . "Self-induced," said Kostoglotov, laying aside his book. He waved his hands, fingers splayed, keeping his leg in the same guitar-like pose. "That means that suddenly for some unexplained reason the tumor starts off in the opposite direction! It gets smaller, resolves and finally disappears! See?" They were all silent, gaping at the fairy tale. That a tumor, one's own tumor, the destructive tumor which had mangled one's whole life, should suddenly drain away, dry up and die by itself?

They were all silent . . . it was only gloomy Podduyev who made his bed creak and, with a hopeless and obstinate expression on his face, croaked out, "I suppose for that you need to have . . . a clear conscience."

These lines are from *Cancer Ward,* by Aleksandr Solzhenitsyn. "A clear conscience," he writes, is the secret. Not a "pure" conscience, not a perfectly virtuous life. That would be too difficult in so little time. It's just about acquiring a little "lifting of the spirit" that will allow you to look at your personal history, both past and present, with a lucid view (without limits, taboos, or judgment). This is the true therapeutic goal of the fifth tool for health—Delta Psychology: to help you have a clearer conscience so you can open wide the door to your path to healing.

In rare cases, this door can lead to an incredible shortcut: spontaneous, self-induced healing. It's impossible to explain this with our current state of scientific knowledge. It goes beyond the framework of this book. But it remains a great ray of hope for our unconscious: the body, in certain circumstances, can express all the power of its healing energies.

You understand by now that the therapeutic aim of Delta Medicine is very different from that of Western medicine, but completely complementary. It's about stimulating our vitality, our healing forces, and, above all, our capability for self-healing. It's about rebalancing and reinforcing our biological terrain. To attain this objective we have already presented you with several tools. There remains one that is special, more personal, and more subtle, but incredibly effective: Delta Psychology.

If Delta Relaxation is aimed at calming and rebalancing your mental state (your ideas, thoughts, nervous system), Delta Psychology strives to harmonize your neuroemotional system (your fears, joys, griefs, regrets, grudges).

DELTA PSYCHOLOGY AND PSYCHOTHERAPY

Before diving in to the subject, I should make it clear that Delta Psychology isn't a psychotherapeutic tool. These exercises do not take the place of psychological or psychiatric help, or psychotherapeutic techniques, whether verbal, behavioral, cognitive, or mind-body. The purpose of Delta Psychology's ritual and symbolic gestures is only to help you make progress up to the present, to better manage your emotional equilibrium.

Keep this in mind: if you are already in therapy (support group, behavioral, or psychoanalytic), you can ask your therapist to integrate this emotional tool for health into your counseling routine. You can also use the tool on your own as personal work. Let your intuition speak to enlarge your dialogue space. These acts may also give you the impetus to consult a therapist if you have not yet done so and feel the need.

Just as Delta Medicine is at the service of traditional medicine, Delta Psychology is at the service of all the techniques belonging to the mental sphere. Delta Psychology doesn't claim to resolve all your emotional problems or your unconscious blocks. But it can help you get in touch with your emotions in the present, without clinging to a more or less painful past that undermines your capacity for healing. The more that painful emotions are deeply buried in the past, the greater the risk that they'll resurface in the form of real psychological, nervous, or physical problems (that is, suffering). This is especially true during moments of emotional shock or pressure tied to stress (when the forces of our conscious personality are weakened and easily overwhelmed by painful pressure from our unconscious).

TAKING ACTION WITHOUT MOVING A MUSCLE

This final tool of Delta Medicine helps patients pull themselves out of a cycle of often obsessive black thoughts, provoked by the announcement of a serious illness. Delta Psychology also constitutes a kind of liaison between the different Delta techniques, a luminous, reassuring, and calming backdrop. It works through a process of symbolic acts, well known in many contemporary therapeutic modalities (behavioral therapies, in particular), but too rarely included in medical regimens in hospitals. For several years now, many Canadian schools of neuroscience have integrated psychological modalities as an adjunct to traditional medicine. Scientists now have at their disposal studies and both enceph-alographic images and MRIs that clearly show the cerebral impact of these rhythmic and symbolic techniques (rituals).

A specific branch of neuroscience, whose practitioners focus on the rehabilitation of people who are seriously injured, clearly shows that when people learn to execute a particular gesture (no matter what it is) and when they assimilate this gesture in their repertoire of movements, you can see on an encephalogram a specific area of the brain stimulated each time they repeat the movement under the same conditions. But, in a startling discovery, if another person performs the same gesture in front of the patient, the same area of the brain is stimulated. So seeing the gesture produces the same neurocerebral alert as performing the ges-ture itself. (See appendix 3 for more details on this discovery.)

This can explain, in part, the real therapeutic impact of ritual acts in ethnomedicine (traditional, ancestral medicine practiced by sha-mans). Without actually moving, we can make our nervous and neuro-muscular system work as if we were in motion.

It turns out that by stimulating the neurophysiological pathways involved in an action like movement, we also stimulate symbolic and emotional correlates to that movement. So a particular movement might conjure up thoughts of fear or anger, while another movement might be associated with thoughts of love or peace. These programmed gestures, then, make us "move" on the inside.

Symbolic acts and ritual gestures are to the unconscious what words and speaking are to the conscious mind. These symbolic gestures are done in order to be perceived and understood by the part of us that underlies our conscious thoughts. Freud calls it the unconscious; Jung, the collective unconscious; some spiritual currents, the subtle energetic dimension. The name matters little. Some of these symbolic gestures might seem infantile, innocent, or even incomprehensible to our thinking brain, which is objective and intelligent. But they are perceived as essential by our emotional brain, which is intuitive and subjective. A very simple, colorful example: Placing our right hand open on the chest at heart level is perceived by the emotional unconscious of all of us around the planet as a sign of peace when the head is held straight and the eyes wide open, but as a sign of suffering when the head is lowered, the hand closed into a fist, and the eyes closed.

THOUGHTS AND EMOTIONS:
TWO DIFFERENT BUT CONVERGING UNIVERSES

We are now at the heart of Delta Psychology, the power of our emotions and their impact on our body as well as on our mental equilibrium and our health. Not only do emotions arise from sensations, feelings, or our state of mind, but they also leave an imprint on our body. They generate a biological reality that we can easily observe, even if, to date, science has not yet pierced the inner workings of that reality. The *virtual* (that is, thoughts) can materialize by way of the *real* (our body's responses) when it is touched by the magic wand of our emotions.

While Delta Relaxation, which we focused on in the previous chapter, was principally based on mental imagery—programmed and directed forms of thought—Delta Psychology is essentially aimed at our major emotions. Even if the two are closely related, they are different. A thought is conceptual: you can think about the color of your clothes, about the shape of your car, about your children's schoolwork. But these thoughts may have an emotional tint: the red that you wear today stimulates you and awakens joy in you; the new car that you just bought brings you pleasure; the children's schoolwork immerses you in worry. To express itself, an emotion needs support, in the form of a thought, an image, or a memory. It begins with something more vague, impalpable, an unclear sensation. Emotion is like a merging of images and thoughts that we color with what we feel. These feelings plant their roots in the depths of our oldest experiences, in what we perceived (by unrolling the film of our life) as positive or negative, pleasant or unpleasant, joyful or sad.

All these emotional colorations (virtual) translate in the body, by means of the (very real) secretion of pleasure hormones (serotonin, dopamine) or displeasure and stress hormones (adrenaline, cortisol). Thoughts are mental images almost always tinged by emotions, while emotions don't necessarily need the support of clear mental images to come to the fore. (This is the fundamental work of the symbolic, which was central to the thinking of Jung.) But emotions can manifest without the support of a thought, in the form of "instantaneous archaic resurgence"; for example, when a simple scent awakens a feeling of déjà vu without our being able to put our finger on the memory in question. The emotion therefore exists before the thought. The emotion always predominates, in all our life and survival functions, in all our healing energies. A poetic synthesis of this scientific concept is expressed felicitously in the famous quote by French philosopher and mathematician Blaise Pascal: The heart has its reasons that reason cannot know.

Emotions are to the body what light is to the cosmos: a pure energy beyond the living. Indeed, contrary to what we think with our "all-powerful" brain, all our ideas have nervous limits. Our emotions, for their part, are limitless, omnipresent, whether present or past.

THE INFLUENCE OF EMOTIONS ON THE BODY

We can observe the daily imprint of our emotions on the body. But it would take thousands of pages to explain all the processes underlying the relationships between our emotions and their physical manifestations. They travel by cerebral pathways, then neurohormonal and neurovascular pathways. An emotion can provoke cardiac or circulatory acceleration; it can have a sexual expression (especially in men). If it concerns fear, it can prompt spasms and/or nausea. An intense fear can modify the distribution of blood in the body, giving priority to the organs that react in the face of danger (the brain, the muscles). This explains why, depending on the situation, an emotion can make us turn pale (vasoconstriction) or, on the contrary, blush (vasodilation). The almost infinite palette of emotional nuances can influence all our biological systems, all our organs, all the body's functions.

Many medical teams have investigated these issues. One group of doctors even studied the impact of emotions on certain bacterial strains populating our intestinal flora. They discovered that repeated violent emotions (anxiety, anger, hatred, grudges, feelings of guilt) progressively transform the composition of the intestinal flora, giving priority to different strains (those that are either more or less pathogenic), depending on the experiences a person encounters—and the emotions those experiences generate—over a period of serenity or tension.

In the past, before the discovery of antibiotics, some bacteriologists thought that they could improve the mental state of their patients by means of intestinal autovaccinations (created by diluting bacterial strains found in a patient's own digestive tract). During the first half of the twentieth century this technique was even successfully integrated into medical practice. But it was swept away with the arrival of antibiotics that gave a more powerful response to the terrible pandemics of microbial origin that decimated worldwide populations in waves over the course of centuries. (Keep in mind, however, that more than half of the great pandemics were eradicated by the medical miracle of hygiene.)

During the same era, in the sanatoriums where tuberculosis patients were treated (the illness is highly contagious), doctors noticed that among the sanatorium personnel, the most resistant were those who led the healthiest lives on a nutritional level, but especially on an emotional level. This was the case with religious workers, whose lives were frugal on a nutritional level and balanced on an emotional level. They had very little external stress: they didn't have to earn money, climb the ladder of social status, find a life partner, or raise children. And their privileged relationship with divine love contributed to their inner harmony. Many of these religious workers had incredibly high levels of resistance to microbial infections. Some treated two generations of patients. That is, they had fifty years of contact with the germ without contracting the disease, yet all it takes sometimes is a few days of contact with someone who has tuberculosis for a person to become seriously ill.

The study of the emotional dimension of illness is nevertheless not new. We can find traces of these studies in all the great traditional medicines: Hippocrates covered it thoroughly in *Materiae medica,* and in Egyptian, Native American, Chinese, and Indian treatises on traditional medicine, emotions are often associated with certain forms of physical suffering. For example, traditional Chinese medicine associates anger with the energy of the liver, and sadness with the spleen. Everyday language sometimes echoes these connections: *full of bile,* or to make someone's *blood boil.* And in French, the word *spleen* refers to the organ, but it also means a state of chronic sadness.

Because emotional pressures loom ever larger in contemporary society, there is more and more research in universities pertaining to their impact on health. A promising new field of research was even born in the 1980s: psychoneuroimmunology. As its name indicates, this discipline is concerned with the relationships that develop between our emotions, our nervous system, and our immune system (and, by rebound, our hormonal, or endocrine, system). The heads of oncology departments have become increasingly interested in it, to the point of integrating it into their research and in their hospital practice (see the foreword).

DAILY EMOTIONS

The core idea behind Delta Psychology is this: when our emotions are harmonized (or at least calmed and experienced with awareness), they can liberate vital energy that will support our healing forces. I'm not claiming that the simple fact of feeling and integrating our emotions in a more serene manner is enough to cure an illness. But it's clear that painful emotions tied to past events and situations that continue to echo and darken our present life certainly aggravate an illness.

If you have truly decided to do everything you can to help your life balance lean to the side of health (bringing it back over the Delta Point), if you have begun to correct the main imbalances that have until now weighed down on your sick side, you must not, you cannot, neglect this work on emotions. Based on all my years of observation, I would rank this tool of health in first place, if it were easier to practice.

Contemporary Western society gives us access to much more information and many more emotions than our ancestors had. But while our emotional life may be rich and varied, our interpersonal communication is impoverished. Today we can connect with half the planet with one single click, but urban overcrowding and the breakup of the multigenerational family have limited the possibilities of intimate exchange. Friendships have also evolved. They have become more shifting, unstable, and superficial. Added to this is a major retrenchment in religious practice. In the past religion offered an important context for the expression of emotions (I'm thinking especially of the main purpose of Catholic confession and of the pastoral counseling of rabbis, imams, or sages). For all these reasons, we have fewer and fewer occasions to express painful emotions, to sanctify them and integrate them into our experience. Emotional difficulties have always existed, but today we must give them a response of our era. Delta Psychology constitutes a first important step, one of recognition without self-judgment; an open door to a more clear-sighted acceptance of our true, profound identity, beyond our constructed personality—the will for a clearer conscience.

EMOTIONS AND HEALTH

Of course, we can't state that certain emotions alone make us sick. That would be a simplistic shortcut. But depending on the character of these emotions (positive or negative, pleasant or painful, joyful or sad), and depending on the quality of our emotional management (the way we experience them, accept or reject them, express or repress them), we can more or less easily find a place within us for a form of inner equilibrium (ideally, for serenity).

In the short or long term, negative emotions, expressed in the wrong way or unexpressed and then repressed (sometimes hidden away), may have a significant biochemical impact. And this impact may end up promoting imbalances in our biological terrain, which can cause genetic weaknesses to emerge. This is why, within some university research programs—notably those in Canada—emotional shocks are listed among the major causes of certain types of cancer.

I personally find this correlation a bit too direct and superficial, as are all the scientific shortcuts that tend to associate the appearance of cancer with one single origin: cancer and nutrition, cancer and stress, cancer and emotional upheaval. But I do think that our emotions are largely worth including among the number of lifestyle factors that can contribute to the deconstruction of cancers and autoimmune or degenerative diseases.

Countless clinical observations can help us understand why a fair number of doctors have integrated questions on the emotional life of their patients into their examinations. And it's not uncommon to discover that a case of multiple sclerosis began after a period of serious problems, or that a case of cancer followed a serious accident, a difficult time of grieving, or another destabilizing event (divorce, unemployment). In short, that emotional period may be the trigger, but it's not the only cause.

LIFE: KINGDOM OF INEQUALITIES?

We are not all born equal from a health standpoint—far from it. Just as some people are born into material wealth and others into poverty, there are those who come into the world with a robust state of health while others inherit "genetic baggage" much heavier to carry. There are those endowed from the beginning with an emotional flexibility greater than that of others. It appears to be a great injustice that we can do nothing about. Life sometimes seems like the kingdom of inequalities. But it's also the kingdom of motivation and hope, because there are now valuable tools that help us to compensate for and sometimes level these numerous inequalities. Just as you can often overcome social inequality by working hard, you can reinforce your body and overcome the pitfalls of a naturally weaker biological terrain by working with perseverance on health and healing energies.

We have no say over the distribution of our organic weaknesses. Our organs secretly have predispositions for health or illness, strength or weakness, from birth (and even before). For some, years of repeated major imbalances are not enough to cause the organic weakness inscribed in the Weak Points chapter of our life book to express them-selves. But for others, these weaknesses will see the light of day in spite of a much healthier lifestyle.

We all know people who smoke their entire life, drink alcohol regularly, eat rich food, and never play sports, yet nevertheless live to one hundred without ever having any health problems. These people have at their disposal robust health beyond the norm. All we can say is, Good for those who enjoy this luck! But we don't harbor any illusions; these cases are definitely the exception. We're not going to abandon any chance of fortifying our own health, of supporting it and sheltering it from problems as much as possible, just because some people have an exceptional genetic constitution.

And the blueprint for our genetic strengths and weaknesses is still rel-atively vague. So in the absence of precise information about our organic strengths and weaknesses, it's wise to integrate the approaches of Delta Medicine, and other preventive medicine regimens, into our daily life.

OUR THREE FUNDAMENTAL EMOTIONS

When we talk about emotions, we are, in reality, referring to three different emotional domains. First there is stress (or, more precisely, an excess of stress) and negative thoughts (associated with unpleasant sensations-emotions); we discussed this in the preceding chapter. Then there are all the emotions related to the way in which we identify ourselves in relation to our parents' desires and expectations, the place that we occupy in the family lineage (with its heavy weight of tradition). This is the vast domain of transgenerational emotions and imprints. Finally, there are personal and interpersonal emotions (with the construction of our social personality). It is this last group that Delta Psychology is concerned with, because these are the most active emotions, and often the easiest to access.

The palette of these emotions is very large, both in nature and in intensity. Emotions can run from the smallest trace of anger to the most ferocious hatred; from slight remorse to the most paralyzing guilt; from superficial enjoyment to the utmost joy. We experience these emotions according to the life we live, the relationships we maintain, and what we experienced during childhood (intimately mixed with the heavy transgenerational baggage). The body expresses all these emotions in its own way. Yet in spite of their incredible richness of expression, emotions can be organized into three categories, corresponding to the three great fundamental emotions: fear, resentment, and guilt.

Fear is closely linked to the very fact of being alive. It is the urge to survive, nestled inside each of our cells, that pushes us to stay alive at any cost. In this preservation instinct, all forms of fear take root, from the simple, fleeting fright to absolute terror. In the chapters on Delta Breathing and Delta Relaxation, we already covered the anxiety that seizes patients upon the announcement of a serious illness, especially cancer. The instinct to survive resonates within them, pushing them, at worst, to deny a reality that is too difficult to accept. At best, it makes them fight and use everything in their power to get through it. Delta Breathing is an effective weapon in fighting against the energy of fear, not to destroy it (that's impossible), but to transform it into a calmer, more positive energy.

Delta Psychology is also closely allied with two other fundamental emotions, much more interconnected than you'd think at first. Resentment and guilt are two related energies that are highly disturbing and destructive. Like other emotions, they have an intensity that varies according to individuals and their personal history. The former can run from a superficial little grudge to the most tenacious anger or hatred; the latter can go from simple, slight regret to shame or a permanent feeling of lack of value. Each case has a common trajectory: resentment consists of negative energies that we direct at others, while with guilt, we direct these negative energies onto ourself. The goal of Delta Psychology is to rebalance these two destabilizing and extremely destructive emotions.

RESENTMENT AND GUILT: TWO INTIMATE POISONS

Resentment and guilt use the support of thoughts, of course, but they also draw from much deeper layers that escape our conscious mind. This is why the work on conscious thought is not enough to defuse these two "intimate poisons." We must find a way to reach the strata below the surface of our being. Delta Psychology accomplishes this by way of symbolic acts. (Ritual acts and symbolism are to the unconscious what words and speech are to the conscious.) I'm referring here to simple techniques, often based on writing, that always respect both individual personality and ethics.

These gestures have an impact that is much stronger because they do not play a part in our everyday attitudes. In our daily life we have access to an "emotional management motor" that uses our habits, our life reflexes, to mask our disturbing emotions (imprinting them as a blockage or a dangerous imbalance in our unconscious). Symbolic and ritual acts are there to short-circuit these habits. In many cases the work helps us to find a new form of serenity. And when emotions are too painful, the symbolic work lets us at least identify the origin of these disturbances and make the always healthy decision of going to seek help from a counselor or therapist. Keep in mind that when I talk about *resentment,* this emotion symbolizes all the negative (weakening) energies of anger directed toward others—violence, hatred, jealousy. Likewise, when I talk about *guilt,* this emotion symbolizes all the negative (weakening) energies of anger directed toward ourself—shame and perpetual self-criticism, lack of self-worth, physical or mental stain, a sense of not being good enough, and various other dysmorphophobias. (The term *dysmorphophobias* refers to disproportionate, and therefore pathological, mental fixations on a part of the body that disturbs an individual.)

THE ROLE OF DELTA PSYCHOLOGY

Of course, simple symbolic acts cannot, by themselves, resolve conflicts whose resonance has registered deeply within us. For that there are effective psychotherapeutic techniques adapted to different types of internal suffering.

Delta Psychology simply offers to help you maintain a more serene relationship with these disturbing emotions, to be able to look them in the face so that they stop sapping your precious vital energy. This energy could be feeding your healing capacities if it weren't engulfed in conflicts belonging to the past, playing on a repeating loop. At the present moment, you need all your energy to deconstruct your illness. Certain emotional conflicts play an integral role in your antihealth imbalances. The symbolic acts of Delta Psychology are aimed specifically at them.

Being able to think about these conflicts, these relationship problems, with a bit more serenity will liberate a good part of this healing energy. If the vague but weighty image of these emotional conflicts disturbs you, it's because they're buried deep inside, sometimes concealed, or even denied. And this negation always consumes a lot of energy, on a psychological and mental level, as well as a physical level.

To summarize: A person has hurt you, betrayed you, wounded you, leading to resentment. You hold a grudge against that person. Or a parallel scenario: You have deeply hurt someone and you nourish a great sense of guilt as a result of it. In each case, this event, which is rooted in the past, mobilizes, consumes, and engulfs part of the vitality you need in the present. To dispel these deleterious emotions, you must detach yourself from this past to reclaim all that energy in the present. As Dr. Wayne W. Dyer says in *10 Secrets of Success and Inner Peace*:

> To live with guilt (or resentment) is to use up your present moments being immobilized over what has already transpired. No amount of guilt will ever undo what's been done. . . . Releasing guilt is like removing a huge weight from your shoulders. . . . You empower yourself with love and respect, letting go of standards of perfection and refusing to use up the precious currency of your life, the now.

Dr. Dyer knows exactly what he's talking about. A doctor of psychology and a renowned psychotherapist, he has devoted his life to the study of emotions and their impact on health.

Releasing resentment or guilt doesn't involve "forgiving" (someone else or yourself), at least not in the Judeo-Christian or Buddhist sense of the term. It's not about absolving anyone of blame, whether the hurtful act was committed by you (guilt) or by someone else (resentment). True forgiveness doesn't involve a decision. It doesn't happen by waving the magic wand of conscious will. Nevertheless, the ritual gestures of Delta Psychology can help you activate the intention, the will, or even the simple desire within you to recapture this vital energy that has been sapped in a sterile and useless way by the memory of a hurtful event that belongs in the past. And you'll be doing this precisely at the moment when you really need it in your present life to nurture your healing forces. These symbolic gestures don't erase what happened in the past, but they help bring back to the present the energy that is uselessly tied up in feelings of resentment or guilt. The energy that was dead, because it was useless, becomes once again living, because it's available. (As an aside: this doesn't preclude, in some cases, the need for your emotions to be calmed through psychotherapy.)

Whatever has already happened belongs to the past and it's no longer possible to change that. But what belongs to the future has not yet come to pass, and nobody can predict from which thread the cloth of our life will be woven. Between the past and the future, we live in a perpetually moving present, like a point observed from above that moves along a trajectory. But it is this point that we must concentrate on, because for whatever steadiness or movement there is, it is only here, in the present, that we have the power to act. It is in this present moment that we are sick. But, above all, it is in this moment that we are conscious agents of each moment of life. And it is in this present moment that we are therefore able to modify some of our habits in a way that favorably influences the oscillations of our life balance.

EXPRESSING OUR WISH TO PARDON

You may wonder what I mean by *ritual act* or *symbolic act*. I'm talking about a very real act, but one that reaches the level of the virtual; it's an act that is simple for your conscious brain to understand and accomplish, but also has the valuable ability to deliver a perceptible message to the unconscious.

One part of the symbolic act of Delta Psychology will consist of a "wish to pardon," in the sense of striving for inner peace, that your unconscious will hear, understand, and integrate. This doesn't mean that the emotional pardon will be granted in one fell swoop, like magic. A true pardon takes time. If one day it does occur, it will give you total liberation, which will be very beneficial for you. But when you are suffering from cancer, time is of the essence. You don't have the time to wait for a pardon. Yet you'll discover that it's always possible to start by expressing your wish to pardon to your unconscious, to reclaim some of the emotional energy that you need immediately. The essence of this major idea of psychology is perfectly summarized in the famous sermon by Martin Luther King Jr.: "Forgiveness does not mean ignoring what has been done or putting a false label on an evil act. It means, rather, that the evil act no longer remains as a barrier to the relationship." This is what you must understand and apply: this voluntary step that you take is going to bring down an emotional barrier that is holding captive a valuable part of your life energy. It is a courageous act that will strengthen your sense of self-worth. This is both the practical and powerful aspect of the technique.

The first thing you'll do is connect yourself with this wish* to pardon. You're going to make a mental image out of it and formulate it as follows: Yes, I want to make peace with the emotions that make me suffer. Yes, I want to liberate myself from this resentment or this guilt that rules me.

There is an excellent reason for this. Resentment feeds on the desire for revenge: you want to make the person who hurt you suffer, to pay him back for inflicting that pain. But in doing this, you're the only one who's suffering. The other person, the guilty party, is unaware of this obsessive wish that troubles you so. What a waste!

On the other hand, by formalizing your wish to pardon, you don't absolve the other of the fault; rather, you begin to free yourself of a very weighty emotional and mental burden.

It works the same way with guilt. If the feeling of guilt is essential because it makes us conscious of good and evil, of justice and injustice, chronic guilt has no emotional utility whatsoever. It does no good to the person you've hurt; all it does is haunt you, trouble you, in a sterile dynamic that only harms you.

The wish to pardon another, the wish to pardon oneself—these are the first two symbolic keys of Delta Psychology. As an aside, note that these liberated emotional energies can be made available for a "restoring act" toward the injured person or a reopening of dialogue (real if the person is still alive; virtual if he or she is deceased) with the person who made you suffer.

---

*If the word *wish* seems too strong for you, try *option to pardon* or *pardon technique* to progressively calm these negative energies held captive in your unconscious. These truly unconscious energies do us very real harm, albeit involuntary.

DELTA PSYCHOLOGY IN PRACTICE

Now you're ready to start. The first step consists of asking yourself what resentments you're holding on to (even if it's for a very long time, or buried down deep), and what guilts you feed (even if it's for acts that you're not responsible for but you would have wanted to avoid). Take the time necessary to let your memories come to the surface and explore them.

For some people, the exercise is obvious: from the very first moment, painful or embarrassing memories are accessible. For others, the progression takes longer. But I can tell you from experience that never has a patient remained blocked and unable to identify a few tenacious grudges or a few secret feelings of guilt.

Some advice to guide you: Think about traumatizing experiences, injustices inflicted on you, past suffering. Then return to memories of your mistakes, your errors (or what you could identify as such), your regrets, episodes from your life that you would prefer to erase because they cause a wave of remorse to rise within you. Consciously and calmly think about that. For once, no one is going to judge you or lecture you.

Many people will see these Delta Psychology exercises as an opportunity to talk to their parents or to those close to them. This is a possibility; the relationships we have maintained with our parents, from our first moment of existence, are imprinted deeply within us, in the deepest layers of our being. Even those who were loved, respected, or pampered have suffered involuntary injustices or were painfully misjudged by their mother or father. In such a situation, it can be hard to direct reproaches at our parents, who have proved their love by bringing us into this world and nurturing us to adulthood. That doesn't stop the wounds from being registered within us, just because our sense of morality and logic forbids us from formulating reproaches, or even sometimes from feeling the effects of them.

This exercise will proceed "between you and you," between you and the unconscious of the world, without anyone outside looking in. For once, you can set aside the limits habitually imposed by society, ethics, education, or religion. For once, you can thoroughly investigate how you think and feel without limiting yourself in any way. You can feel perfectly at ease. You're activating a tool to improve your health, and perhaps even facilitating your healing.

To achieve this, you must fully love yourself, if only for just a few moments. This is what will allow you to express yourself without limits or inhibitions, swimming against the current of your upbringing and your "emotional formatting." Forget for a moment all your will to pardon or excuse yourself. Let your anger, hatred, and darkest feelings run freely. Become aware of all these rough "cries of the heart" lying dormant deep within you. Don't be afraid to look them in the face. What follows will help you make peace with them.

The first ritual exercise is based on writing. Have faith in your pen. This isn't about writing well or making up nice turns of phrase. Nobody will be judging your style. You only have to make sure that your pen encounters no filters or censorship. The writing will help you to find all the violence (and pain) of your hidden emotions, even the most shameful. In almost all cases, the wound is one of love (too much, not enough, badly given) that is hidden behind these wounds to the spirit. And it's this energy of wounded love that Delta Psychology will help you reclaim to better support your natural healing forces.

▲ The Writing Phase

According to Paulo Coelho, author of *Maktub:* "The simple fact of writing helps us to organize our thoughts and see more clearly what is in our surroundings. A paper and pen perform miracles—they alleviate pain, make dreams come true and summon lost hope. The word has power." Let's use the power of the word to our benefit, and to the benefit of our health.

When you feel ready, you can start "filing": organize your grudges and guilts by order of importance so that you determine the three most important, those that have affected you the most, preoccupied you the most, and hurt you the most.

- Each of these painful emotions is connected to a central person who hurt you or whom you have hurt. Clearly identify each of those people.

- Take three notebooks (or two or one, if there are only one or two painful emotions within you; if you've identified more, you can deal with the additional people after this first session of Delta Psychology is completed).

- On the first page of each notebook, write the name of one of the people. If possible, attach a photo of the person underneath the name.

- If you only know the first name, write that. And if you don't even know the first name, write a sentence that represents that person. For example, "The person I hit with my car, on such-and-such a day, at such and-such a place."

- It's possible that you'll only identify one painful emotion, one event, or one person. Then begin with one notebook. If, over the course of writing, other emotions or other central people surface, you can use other notebooks.

- Next, for three days, spend a moment each morning looking at each name and allow the emotions attached to this person to arise within you. Three to five minutes is enough. You can choose to listen to music that you connect with this person or your shared experiences to help you with this.

- On the morning of the fourth day, you will begin to write all the emotions you feel toward each person in the corresponding notebooks. Whether you feel resentment or guilt, let the tide of thoughts and sensations gush forth. It doesn't matter if you're disrespectful, crude, or insulting. If it has to do with one of your faults, let the self-deprecation and reproaches flow freely, even if they're violent. Don't censor yourself. While you're writing, allow yourself to be the person you would have loved to have been in the past, at the moment when the painful memory took place. Let the emotions that have remained all these years inside your painful memories emerge.

- In the evening, reread what you wrote in the morning and add whatever seems important to you. The next morning, continue.

■ You will write and rewrite this way, several times in a row. For some, it only takes a few days. For others, it takes a few weeks.* It doesn't matter. There will come a time when you feel deep down inside you that all the vicious emotions have left. Then you will know, within your body and mind, that you have arrived at the very end of this exercise.

■ You can, at your convenience, fill several notebooks successively, or stick with one and wait until you've finished it to start another. But be careful: this phase of fundamental writing can hide an emotional snare—discouragement, excess emotion, or, worse, disgust at what you've done or what you've suffered, or at who you now are as you face this report. If a person adds the weighty and often devaluing context of illness, the overall picture can seem pretty dark, perhaps even crushing. You should immediately curb this impulse, which comes from your ego and damaged emotions, and impose a lively, positive, and, above all, very real thought: That's not all you are. You are not just an upset body and sterile emotions. You are not just the sum of your resentments, guilts, and errors. You are also fundamentally a luminous being, with valuable qualities, experiences, and life successes. Your body may be weakened or suffering, but you're alive. You may have lost your way, or suffered physical and moral wounds head-on; you may have felt fear, jealousy, resentment, hatred, or a dozen guilty feelings gnawing at you (both real and imaginary). But never, ever forget that none of that is you. Now you have the will and the courage to walk away from these weighty energies and become freer, more at peace, more luminous, and better healed.

This essential truth leaves no more room for discouragement, impatience, or disgust. This essential truth is just the first step in your new momentum to heal.

At this stage, you may start to feel a slight sense of relief and calm.

---

*One of my patients took three years to write the text, but that was a unique case in my practice.

This is a sign that you have finally arrived at the end of the first step. You have moved from a pure dialogue of the mind (thoughts, images) to the enthusiasm of a dialogue of the heart (emotions).

▲ The Symbolic Phrase

You are now going to enter the symbolic phase (and phrase!) of the work. We have developed this practice with psychologists and psychotherapists in order to begin to address and repair your emotional disorders. The goal of this step is to create the desire within you to forgive or to forgive yourself. To do this, you are going to use a symbolic phrase that will help you establish a dialogue with yourself, all the way to the depths of your unconscious, whether the people involved are alive or not (and even if you don't know whether they're alive or not). This is one of the great strengths of Delta Psychology. Many people remain blocked for years, or almost their entire life, by negative emotions they don't succeed in uprooting because those involved in the conflict are deceased. But in both your unconscious and the world's unconscious, time and death do not exist. You must use the emotional strength of this new space for dialogue to your benefit.

- Once you have the feeling that you have put everything on paper and that you've arrived at the end of what you have to say, you will find that you have a totally different inner energy. You have moved from the energy of the mind to the energy of the heart.
- You will benefit from this different inner state and write in your notebook a symbolic phrase after the reproaches or excuses. Something like the following:

> Dear [name of the person as it appears on the first page of your notebook],
> Today I'm [your current age] years old. As an adult who is conscious of my feelings, I want to pardon you for what you have done to me.

Or:

Dear [name of the person as it appears on the first page of your notebook],

Today I'm [your current age] years old. As an adult who is conscious of what I've done to you, I am sorry, and ask that you please accept my apologies and pardon me.

■ You can follow that model, or construct a similar sentence that works better for you, one that resonates more clearly within you.

In this way, you address the person involved (dad, mom, brother, or sister; Peter, Paul, Jack, or Mary), citing your current age and positioning yourself as the adult that you've become and not the child, adolescent, or young adult who was hurt, or who inflicted harm, in the past. We may all succeed at becoming adults on a social level, but not necessarily on an emotional level. During this phase, you tell yourself that your life is no longer determined by how others perceive you, that you detach yourself from social and educational imprints, and that you finally know who you are.

Of course, you'll express this phase of pardons or excuses with words that your conscious thoughts have formulated. But the fact of writing it more strongly imprints your desire to pardon or apologize, all the way to the deepest layers of your being, to a place where you can tame your suffering.

▲ Acts of Freedom

We've arrived at the last step in this ritual and symbolic process. You are now going to free yourself from what you have unearthed from your past, what you expressed and released in the two previous exercises. To do this, you're going to perform a little ritual inspired by some practices used in traditional medicine. Traces of it can be found in regions throughout the world and across millennia. Don't worry: you're not going to enter a trance or dance all night around a fire. This practical act is much simpler and within everyone's reach, but it's very powerful.

You'll be able to choose your freedom ritual depending on whether you're introverted or extroverted. Read carefully and to the end of the two scenarios, and then choose one, following your intuition. You'll definitely make the right choice. At this stage, have confidence in yourself and your feelings.

These two symbolic practices are equivalent in terms of effectiveness and both work on the unconscious. The first one calls on more of an imaginative energy (poetic, artistic, musical). The second is more active (grounded, organized, animal). I repeat, both are good; what's important is to choose one and do it.

Liberation Protocol #1: Imaginative Energy

You have just written the essence of your emotional reality with courage, perseverance, and lucidity. And you have done so face-to-face with the person key to your personal suffering.

You have consciously written your symbolic wish to pardon another (resentment) or yourself (guilt). Perfect! You have taken a big step, but this step is still too intellectual. You must take it deeper, to the energy of your heart, your emotions, to the hidden layers of your profound emotions.

Writing thoughts and prose (your text as it is now) has essentially made your left brain work (it's not neurologically as precise and separated as that, but we'll adopt this simplified left brain–right brain explanation as an easy way for you to envision what we're doing). You now need to make your right brain work, with the same emotional ideas.

How does this work? First of all, the scientific observation of electroencephalograms and MRIs of individuals reading prose or poetry in a controlled environment shows that the rhythm, rhymes, and music of words in a poem tend to activate the brain's right hemisphere. On the second or third reading of a poem, this becomes easily observable, because the first reading is still oriented toward deciphering the words (left brain), and this interferes with the inherent musicality of the words (right brain).

Without comparing yourself to Rimbaud, Ginsberg, or Shakespeare, you will create your own emotional music. You will now "poeticize" your past sufferings. And by doing this, you will overcome them. You'll break down the walls that have held your energy captive.

■ Reread several times out loud the first text in your notebook.

■ Then from this base, start composing a poetic summary, with strong rhymes (musicality is primordial). Here are two brief examples. They may seem a bit like caricatures, but they're models that can be followed (by adapting them, of course, to your own emotional history and by expanding them beyond one stanza, if needed):

> Dear Mom,
>> When my brother was born,
>> You left me forlorn.
>> And your love for me
>> Was gone, I could see.

Or even:

> Dear John,
>> You I loved with all my heart,
>> But you the jerk tore me apart.
>> I fulfilled your wishes every day,
>> But you made a new life, far away.

■ Don't hold back. Create. Create your poem without ideological or linguistic taboos. Impose no limits on your words, so that you can fully express your pain and hurt. Re-create your story, your suffering. Roll out the laughter and tears of pain and joy, using the music of words. You can write one to two pages. This is usually enough. But if the exercise inspires you, amuses you, relaxes you, keep going. Write ten pages, if you'd like!

Some patients (who generously let me read what they wrote) have created sublime poems, while other poems were the worst of the worst (the opinion was unanimous, expressed with a sense of humor and laughter). But everyone, without exception, knew how to make music from the heart.

That's the goal. That's the sign that you've completely succeeded at this liberation protocol. So be daring and make this exercise your own.

- The final phase of this exercise is very simple: once you've finished your poem, start by burning all the pages of the base text (what you wrote in prose) in a big pot, placed in your kitchen sink so that you run no risk of setting a fire (you must remain prudent and practical, even in the symbolic and virtual world).

- Next, carefully memorize your poem (the magic of words). Once you're certain that you know it inside and out (this may take up to two weeks), burn your poem, too (once again, safely!).

- Some of my patients decided to put their poem to the tune of their choice. They found this even more powerful and liberating. I've taken their remarks and observations into account and now offer this creative option to all my patients.

- From now on, each time you think about this person, this situation, and this suffering, the poem will come back to you (in words or as a song). And the emotional recollection will no longer occur in your left brain (the side of mind games and self-criticism), but rather in your right brain (the side of emotions, now calm). You'll reclaim your valuable healing energies, for the present, your current life, here where you really need it.

It's up to you to play, to create, and to improvise. I repeat: no limits, no holding back. This is your personal challenge as a way to heal.

Liberation Protocol #2: Active Energy

Here is the more grounded, Jungian scenario. It reflects some of the hypotheses related to the symbolic formulated by psychoanalyst Carl Gustav Jung, a disciple and dissident of Freud (see appendix 2).

Ritual Act of Purification

- Take a large pot that you can burn paper in without any danger. Place the pot in the kitchen sink with the faucet close at hand, just in case.

- Begin by tearing the pages you've written out of the notebook, then read them out loud. If the text you've written is too long, read a summary of it that covers the essence of what you've written.

- Finish your reading with the pardon or excuse phrase, repeating it three times out loud, very slowly.
- Then burn the notebook's pages in the pot, along with the first page, where the name and perhaps the photo of the person appear.

Ritual Act of Dissolution and Pacification

- Once you have finished all this burning and everything has cooled completely, find a piece of ground where you can bury the ashes. Ideally, this will be in your yard, but you can also use a window box on your balcony or a small spot out in nature.
- Take a jar of honey, a living plant, and a small hand trowel (if you don't own one, a large, stainless-steel spoon will work).
- Dig a small hole in the ground (about eight to twelve inches deep), dump the ashes in it, and then pour one quarter of the jar of honey on top of it. Cover with dirt.*

Symbolic Act of Transmutation

- Plant the living plant on top of the buried ashes and honey, where it can take nourishment from the dirt, ashes, and honey to grow. The death of the past (the ashes) will give birth to a new, positive, living energy in the present. For you, it is the promise of newfound peace and vitality.

Does this ritual seem strange, or even a tad ridiculous? You absolutely must not linger on this judgment expressed by your logical mind. These gestures have powerful, ancestral, and symbolic meanings that speak not only to the logic of the heart but also to our collective history, whose roots run deep into humanity's most distant past.

Fire plays a part in all rituals of purification. The act of pouring honey on the ashes makes soothing sweetness—a maternal symbol of gentleness and peace—flow over what remains of your suffering. (An

---

*This refined symbolic ritual resulted after many discussions with filmmaker Alejandro Jodorowsky and actress and writer Marianne Costa, who have collaborated on books and workshops about spirituality and psychogenealogy.

aside: Some people prefer to use milk for ritual acts related to a mother, a child, a sister, or a brother. Don't hesitate to do this if the symbolism of milk resonates more strongly for you than honey on an emotional level.) And when you plant a seedling in this emotionally charged ground, you reach the ultimate goal of all transmutation: to nourish a living entity (the plant) in the present, with the transmuted remains of your past suffering; to nourish your healing with the reclaimed and transmuted energy of your past suffering.

PRACTICAL SUMMARY

Choose one of the two ritual liberation paths, and, above all, do not let your conscious thoughts judge you while you execute these rituals.

We've offered them based on what we've learned from our contact with patients. Remember that your intellectual logic is very different from your emotional logic. If you agree to set aside your conscious thoughts for a few minutes (the part of your mind that judges, comments, and buzzes nonstop in your head, and that affixes labels on the smallest of your actions), you will let these simple, symbolic acts fulfill their role: to bring back to the present the energies imprisoned in the past in order to make them available for your healing process.

To do that, all you have to do is concentrate on what you have to accomplish, on each one of your words, on each one of your gestures. Have total faith in this tool of mind-body medicine. You've already noticed to what extent emotions respond to rules that have nothing to do with conscious or logical thinking. Remember: a simple scent, a few notes of a song, or the sight of an object can be enough to awaken a powerful emotion in you, and at times you may not even know where that emotion comes from. I suggest that you put these emotional resonances to use for your health, by way of these symbolic exercises of Delta Psychology.

I must emphasize, once again, that these gestures are no substitute for actual psychotherapeutic work or psychoanalysis. So if you feel the need to get psychological help, don't hesitate to do so. These are just tools from practical research in the neurosciences and mind-body medicine that are designed to calm and reinvigorate the neuroemotional system. They readjust particular energies that are prisoners of the past to allow for a new, more harmonious distribution of your feelings (and your healing efforts) in the present.

I will once again use the example of a car. This time the car is equipped with a GPS. If its satellite reference marks are badly calibrated by only a few degrees when it's made, it will never lead you too far off course for short trips. But if you travel a couple hundred miles, (from New York to Washington, D.C., for example), this very slight discrepancy will end up producing enough of an accumulated error effect to send you to Bethesda, Maryland (located six miles to the east).

Likewise, an emotional wound that seems to be minor (or is carefully blocked in your unconscious) can, over the years, contribute to building within you the foundations of true suffering—first emotional, then relational, and finally physical (that is, a disease).

Conversely, a series of ritual acts, calming and infused with symbolic messages, can provoke big rebalancing therapeutic effects within you (a recalibration of your emotional GPS), above all if it is done in synergy with the other health practices.

You now have at your disposal the five tools for health, offered by the complete Delta Medicine program. They'll be within reach every day, until they're in the palm of your hand. That's the true goal of this book.

"You cannot teach a man anything. You can only help him discover it within himself," the great physicist and astronomer Galileo said with wisdom. I hope that your inner discoveries have been numerous, surprising, motivating, and, above all, useful to your great life project: to heal!

Key Points

→ Delta Psychology cannot be compared to the work accomplished by numerous forms of psychotherapy. This psychological tool only helps to better manage our emotional equilibrium, and can potentially give us the impetus to consult a therapist if we then feel the need.

→ Delta Psychology helps us come to terms with part of our past emotions and liberate the energy that they imprison. An energy that's lacking in the present is then reclaimed for our healing forces.

→ Delta Psychology can also be very useful for more rapidly banishing the black, obsessive thoughts provoked by illness.

→ Delta Psychology draws on symbolic acts and rituals. These are conscious actions, carried out in the present, that resonate with painful events of the past (often blocked in our unconscious but with a root visible to the conscious mind).

→ All our emotions (virtual) manifest in the body as hormonal secretions (quite real) of pleasure or displeasure that have measurable physiological effects. Their physical reality can prove to be balancing or disturbing, depending on the quality of our emotions and, above all, our ability to manage them.

→ The three most disturbing emotions in terms of health and equilibrium are fear (see the Delta Relaxation chapter), resentment, and guilt.

→ Resentment is a form of violence directed toward others; guilt is a form of violence directed at ourself. These are two intimate poisons. Whatever their origins may be, they uselessly hold energy captive in the past. By liberating this energy, we stimulate our healing forces.

→ Delta Psychology not only erases past sufferings, it also allows us to look at them through the eyes of an adult (not those of a hurt child), and it stimulates a desire to pardon faults committed by others or ourself.

→ The Delta Psychology tool presented here begins with a writing exercise, followed by the personal (intuitive) choice between two ritual, symbolic acts of liberation.

→ Even if the two liberating scenarios offered here may seem ridiculous to the conscious mind, you must put them into practice with a sense of serenity, or even amusement, but, above all else, without judgment. Our ancestral unconscious understands symbolic gestures, rather than everyday words. This unfamiliar emotional access route is one of the strengths of Delta Psychology.

→ Strong negative emotions that have been transmuted into quiet, calm ones in the present are the guarantee of stronger, more vital healing forces, and oftentimes long-lasting health.

AFTERWORD

*First say to yourself what you would be; and then do what
you have to do.*

EPICTETUS, STOIC PHILOSOPHER

Beyond the purely therapeutic medical message of this book, what is the
essence of its human message? Poetically, these are the words that might
have been pronounced by the guardian angel who laid us down in our
cradle for the first time:

> *Never forget that by being born, you came out victorious
>   in the great battle for life.*
> *Don't forget that each day is a gift from life, and you are
>   celebrated with the honors owed to a king or queen.
>   Don't forget that you have the richest, most precious,
>   and marvelously complex kingdom in creation: your
>   body, the guardian of your spirit.*
> *Don't forget to be its protector—respectful, fair, and
>   good.*
> *Don't forget that if some parts of your kingdom
>   rebel (autoimmune diseases), fall into decadence
>   (degenerative diseases), or switch to the side of the*

*enemy (tumors), you nevertheless remain their
uncontested master if you have the will to promptly
reaffirm your authority over your life, your right to
live, and your right to health.*

*Never forget: whatever your worries, your errors, your
fears, your physical and human dramas, you remain
king or queen of your body and your most intimate
cellular equilibrium up to your very last breath.
Think about your time on this planet. Think about
it often and act accordingly. Find the courage,
authority, and life energy within you. Always believe
and accept that you can return to a healthy body and
a harmonious mind.*

As an adult, you should remember these words each night, just before you fall asleep. Then say with strength *what you really want to be,* and each day *do what you really have to do!*

CONCLUSION

As soon as you trust yourself, you will know how to live.
JOHANN WOLFGANG VON GOETHE, *FAUST*

Your body's medicine at the service of the field of medicine may hold wonderful, incredible surprises for you.

Recovery may be for tomorrow, but well-being is for today! This is the first motivating force of Delta Medicine, a medicine of better well-being on a daily basis, a resolutely positive medicine that you can start this very instant, here and now, to put yourself on the road back to health (or to prevent illness from overtaking you).

Little health techniques easily become health practices at the service of all other medical therapies and all your healing processes.

Please allow me one last piece of advice, like a mantra: be curious, read, reread, criticize, or doubt—but try!

Always keep in mind that no one (not even the best of doctors) ever knows enough to be a pessimist. So try, really try! Try one month, just one short month. Try without cheating, without lying to yourself, without lying to me. Try in all good conscience and with consistency. Try these five basic Delta techniques to gently reprogram yourself: breathing, nutrition, detoxification, work on the mind (relaxation), and work on the emotions (psychology).

Experience has proved to me that a month is enough for you to develop a sense of confidence, joy, and inner strength. Enough time to discover new physical and mental strengths in yourself (sometimes unsuspected), to better serve your body and your medical team. Enough time for your life force to help you heal and affirm that you are the true owner of your health. I'm talking here about true health, synonymous with peace and serene certitude; health beyond a simple remission and beyond your fears of relapse; health beyond your former fears and all your illness imprints.

We've arrived together at the end of this voyage. It's been great getting to know you through my words, words chosen with great care. Words to touch your mind and spirit and light the flame of your curiosity, and then spark your motivation. Words to touch your heart and open the door of hope. Finally, words to touch your world of emotions and offer a Delta space of peace and serenity within you.

A book for you, to you, with spaces between my words—blanks that you were able to color with all the infinite nuances of your own personality. This book has become your book: that has been my wish from the first page. It can also become your adventure, and these tools for health are your living forces of healing and recovery.

Perhaps one day soon you'll dare to smile that smile of pride that appears on the faces of those who have arisen victorious from the greatest of challenges: healing!

APPENDIX 1

TEN PRACTICAL HEALTH SUGGESTIONS

Because this book is essentially practical, it may surprise you that these ten suggestions appear as an appendix.

The explanation for this is simple: the carefully organized Delta Medicine program that I offer you is the best of the simplest strategies distilled from all my years of medical experience. More information, suggestions, or recommendations would only dilute the spirit, and in the end weaken the overall effectiveness. I wanted to avoid the temptation of better that can quickly become the enemy of the good.

Nevertheless, I held on to the idea that this book should give you ten additional recommendations just as valuable but of a more general nature, in addition to the program for healing in the main text.

Read them attentively and practice them carefully. They're not techniques or tools for health, but simply practical advice and common sense that can sometimes play a key role in your healing process. The advice has been carefully selected from my thirty years of multidisciplinary investigations into health.

1. QUIT DRINKING ALCOHOL (AT LEAST TEMPORARILY)

Alcohol and cellular problems shouldn't be mixed. Abnormal cells love foods with an elevated glycemic index. It's one of their weaknesses.

Like healthy cells, they need glucose to survive and create their own toxic energy, but they transform it less efficiently. This is why they need more sugar flow. Depriving them of foods and beverages with a high carbohydrate index (red zone foods in the Metabolic Index) weakens them and makes the body stronger. Alcohol has a very high glycemic index. Moreover, it will directly attack the liver and pancreas, and if you're fighting an illness, this is not the time to place stress on these key organs.

So respect this absolute rule for at least six months: no hard liquor of any kind, no cooked wines, such as port or liqueurs, and no beer. The only acceptable exception is a very good glass of red Bordeaux (6–7 ounces) per day, sipped over the course of a meal. All other kinds of liquor will only compromise your healing forces. Forget about drinking for a few months (and resolve to do this without frustration in order to reinforce your healing), until you have returned to a more stable state of health.

2. REDUCE YOUR CONSUMPTION OF TOBACCO

Tobacco and cellular problems don't go well together, either. I'm not only referring to lung and throat cancer, which are directly connected to smoking; I'm talking about all kinds of degenerative diseases.

Quitting smoking is easier said than done—I'm aware of that. The intense stress connected with weaning your body off nicotine and missing the gesture itself of holding a cigarette, or chewing tobacco, can aggravate stress connected to the disease.

You must absolutely avoid the trap of too much willpower. I suggest you use common sense and opt for a happy medium.

- If you're a big smoker (20–40 cigarettes a day), slowly reduce your intake over 30 days until you're smoking just 10 cigarettes a day. Reward yourself for your progress—but not by taking a smoke!
- If you're an average smoker (less than 15 cigarettes a day), reduce

your intake over 30 days until you're smoking just 5 cigarettes a day.

- If you're a light smoker (less than 5 cigarettes a day), make a determined effort to quit completely.

In each case, avoid using nicotine substitutes to help you, such as chewing gum or the nicotine patch. The daily doses are too difficult to regulate and can become toxic, especially for a weakened and unbalanced biological terrain.

To replace cigarettes, I suggest this little holistic secret: buy 250 grams of sweet flag (*Acorus calamus*) at a health food store (it may need to be ordered). This root, which resembles licorice, comes in small pieces about the size of half a hazelnut. It's easy to use: chew a small piece of the plant for ten minutes whenever you want to smoke. It's very effective; the taste may not be terrific, but it's tolerable.

I advise you to quit smoking, not only to protect yourself from the dangers of tobacco but above all to decontaminate your body and give it the breath necessary to mobilize your healing forces. During this period of cutting back, think about having two cups of my special detox mix that you'll find in the Delta Detoxification chapter. A body that is well drained, detoxified, and decontaminated is fully available to welcome all the new energies for healing and recovery.

3. NEVER USE MOTHBALLS, SCENTED CANDLES, OR CHEMICAL AIR FRESHENERS

Too much "progress" has lengthened the list of insidious indoor pollutants. Included in this category are naphthalene mothballs, chemical air fresheners, automatic toilet bowl cleaners, and scented candles made with artificial perfumes. Some products from Eastern Europe and Asia even contain arsenic derivatives that are legal (!) in weak doses. I personally consider them to be very toxic. These chemical substances are not eliminated from the body; they accumulate in the short term and become toxic in the long term. Be vigilant. Carefully read the labels on products, throw out anything that seems suspect, and purify your house with natural incense or an essential oil diffuser (choose pure, organic oils): lavender, thyme, rosemary, eucalyptus. And don't forget that the easiest way to cleanse spaces at home or at work is to open the windows to air them out well several times a day.

4. STOP USING CHEMICAL HAIR COLORING, CHEMICAL DEODORANTS, AND ALUMINUM DISHES AND UTENSILS

These three recommendations may seem unconnected. Yet they have one point in common: they're major sources of internal pollution, notably chemical molecules and heavy and light metals. Their detrimental effects on cellular health are little known to most people, yet dreadful.

Chemical hair coloring contains paraben, resorcine, and ammonium hydroxide. The accumulated effect of these toxic molecules in contact with our scalp is a veritable time bomb. If you want to put all chances to heal on your side, make the effort to give up all permanent hair coloring for several months (six to twelve). This may demand a true effort on your part to give up the aesthetic pleasure, but it will pay off.

Tints sold in health food stores are light in chemical substances but not totally lacking in toxic molecules (with the exception of one or two European brands that are truly 100 percent natural, but don't cover gray well).

If you wish to use henna, choose only products sold in health food stores. Some hennas sold in markets or ethnic stores are called *natural* but are fraudulently reinforced with extremely polluting and toxic lead fixers.

The same points apply to chemical deodorants, and even so-called "natural *and* chemical" deodorants. Mixing extracts from plants with pollutants is a very popular trend among unscrupulous manufacturers. The toxic molecules are different in this case (principally all derivatives from aluminum), but the pollution and cellular damage they cause occur all the same.

Perspiring is a natural and necessary bodily function, crucial for the body's thermal regulation and draining. Never block your perspiration process with antiperspirants. Simply use naturally scented baby wipes several times a day. These ensure both comfort and health.

The last component in toxic metals pollution, both heavy and light: dishes and kitchen utensils made of aluminum. Here again, the principle of precaution is paramount: many studies seem to have established a strong correlation between an excess of certain aluminum ions in the brain and degenerative cerebral illnesses (with Alzheimer's at the top of the list). Other analyses, fewer in number, contradict these results. Don't wait to find out which studies are right. Protect your health by opting for stainless steel, enameled cast iron, or copper.

5. CONSULT (ONCE) YOUR DENTIST

Begin your Delta Medicine program with a visit to your dentist as soon as you can. Cavities, cysts, granulomas (small areas of inflammation), old fillings (mercury pollution), microbial infections, mycoses (fungal infections)—they're all enemies of your cellular health. Ask for a complete checkup and a panoramic x-ray.

Poor dental health doesn't just affect your mouth. It can contaminate (even destroy, in the long term) some of the body's organs, beginning with the heart. (Bacteria from dental granuloma may migrate in the blood and reach the valves of the heart to progressively eat away at them.)

I've had very good experiences with this health practice and very good feedback from all my patients. Free fascia (fibrous connective tissue) and flexible muscular chains make happy organs—stronger, with fewer spasms, and therefore better able to metabolize toxins, neutralize pollutants, and vanquish abnormal cells.

6. CONSULT (ONCE) AN OSTEOPATH

The repeated stress from daily life and the stress of an illness can build up and produce multiple organic, muscular, and nervous tensions. Of course, Delta Breathing and Delta Relaxation have been created to specifically target these problems. But you'll progress more quickly with your healing process by also getting a checkup with a reputable, professional osteopath. When choosing your doctor, take into account the criteria for selection summarized in appendix 3.

7. APPLY THE "PRECAUTION PRINCIPLE" TO ALL ELECTRIC DEVICES!

I've remained in touch with some of the physicians I met when I first began my studies. The consensus among these scientists is clear: the principle of precaution must be applied to all electric or electronic appliances that emit or receive waves.

Here is some practical advice to apply to your daily life in order to limit the risks linked to the use of these devices:

- Never use your cell phone without a headset (not Bluetooth or other wireless devices that promote harmful waves). Use it minimally in your motor vehicle because the interior of a car constitutes a sort of "Faraday cage" that locks in harmful waves.
- Do not leave any electronic device plugged in within your sleeping or relaxation space, even if it's on snooze. This advice holds equally true for Wi-Fi waves emitted by all devices that provide Internet access.
- You can use a microwave oven to reheat food, but not to cook it. In all cases, don't go over 600 watts of power (it will only take a few seconds longer) and wait several minutes before eating microwaved food.
- Never use a microwave oven to defrost foods. Let them defrost in

the refrigerator or at room temperature by taking them out of the freezer in the morning for that afternoon or evening. It's easier on their molecules. In fact, the more quickly a food is defrosted, heated, or cooked, the more its molecular organization is violently agitated, and sometimes irremediably changed. Structural modifications of food are progressively weakening on our organs of digestion and assimilation.

8. WALK!

The best physical activity for reinforcing all your healing energies is walking. It's easy to do and can be adapted to most conditions. Here's an ideal program: first, walk calmly for fifteen minutes, at a strolling pace; then, for the next fifteen minutes walk as quickly as possible. For the last fifteen minutes, adopt an average speed, steady and without exerting yourself.

While walking, always breathe through the nose, pacing your steps to the cadence of your breath: one, two, three steps, I inhale; one, two, three steps, I exhale. Try to concentrate on your breathing and the present moment, observing what's around you and listening to your environment.

The ideal environment for walking is, of course, out in nature. If you live in a city, you can walk in a park or some other green space. Stop to touch nature from time to time: choose a strong, tall tree and place your hands on the trunk, closing your eyes. Concentrate on all its force and power; if you feel the need, ask the tree to support your healing energies. It's a symbolic act, of course, but the positive impact might surpass your expectations.

9. RESPECT YOURSELF

Self-respect is essential to healing. Here are some key ideas to help you maintain your physical and mental health on a daily basis.

- Breathing better is healing better: take breaks often to do Delta Breathing.
- Eating well is healing well: food builds your body. Get to know food better, and cook for yourself if you can.
- Chewing well promotes healing: progressively give yourself this bit of time for your health; it's simple and effective.
- Before campaigning for the ecology of our planet, think about your own cellular ecology. Don't ever forget that your body is your first planet. Do not pollute your body with industrial foods that are too refined, too chemical, too transformed, and too antihealth. Do not allow yourself to be convinced by disrespectful marketing promises: they're easy to spot. I use this infallible strategy: the more I see ads for a product, the less likely I am to buy it.
- Try not to trick yourself: trying to be someone you really aren't consumes large stores of internal energy, both nervous and emotional. In addition, this type of attitude attracts people who aren't meant for you, people with whom you can't maintain just and beneficial relationships.
- Try not to trick others: lies, deceit, and criticism behind someone's back always return to us like a stressful boomerang. This negative behavior nourishes uneasiness, useless conflicts, and feelings of unworthiness. So give yourself a bit of Delta Conscience and don't take part in it!
- Finally, try not to live beyond your means. This is one of the great traps in our consumerist society, and it's one of the greatest sources of stress in contemporary life. So, for at least a few months, try resisting the temptation of buying things; instead, try reusing, renewing, and recycling.

By following these prescriptions, you'll stabilize your interpersonal and material situation. Your health may depend on it. It's definitely worth the effort on your part, and may even revitalize your overall motivation and your healing energies.

10. TRAVEL ALONG THE PATH TO HEALING FOR YOURSELF, FIRST AND FOREMOST

A couple of questions and one last piece of advice that perhaps ought to be at the beginning of this appendix, if not the book itself. You want to heal? You are able to heal? Great! But why? For whom? I can't directly help you with these last two questions. But in my experience, you should know that it absolutely ought to be first of all for yourself.

If you want to win the fight for life (recovery) and you want to become stronger (and happier), you must understand one essential truth: you are the only owner of your terrain (biological, mental, moral), with its weaknesses (diseases), but also all its strengths (healing energies).

Nobody can share your physical or emotional suffering. Nobody can carry the illness of another human being (even if you love that person madly). Illness is a weed whose roots have grown in your terrain, not that of your neighbor. Many people (medical teams, relatives, friends) can help you pull it out. That's the magic of human capability and fraternity. But the origin, the history, and the adventure of your illness and your healing belong to you and you alone. If you understand this and accept it, you will draw incredible strength from it.

That brings us back to the question: Why heal?

This question might seem stupid, indecent, or even disrespectful in view of your suffering. The answer seems obvious: you want to heal to be healthy again, to be able to live. To just live, to be totally alive.

Of course. But what do you really want to do with this newfound health? In this form, the question becomes fundamental and calls for a very personal response that will help speed up your journey along the path to healing. I'd like to be able to help you with this by revealing a very important thought: you can't resolve a problem by preserving the state of mind that created it. Something must change in you so that you're able to discover new responses and new emotional and relational ways of being.

This is valid in countless domains, but it's especially valid for those dealing with cancer. So, in order for your motivation to heal to be complete (completely engaged and completely effective), consider your life each day, gently but clearly. Don't keep your eyes fixed on what you'd like your existence to be, nor on what it would be if you were healed. Look sincerely at what your daily life context is now, where it comes from, and where it's going. Try to go beyond denial and illusions so that your will to heal doesn't remain locked in a dream state, rather than emerging into reality.

The sources of tension and pressure may be ubiquitous: a job that's (too) stressful; a relationship that's (too) one-sided or violent; a rapport with parents that's (too) conflicted; unsatisfactory relations with your own children; frustrations, suffering, intolerable surrounding energies.

You cannot (and you definitely must not) change everything at once. But you can try to make Delta life changes that will provoke a Delta change of spirit.

That's enough. Believe me. In my experience, this is sufficient to help you start the deconstruction of your illness, all the while giving true meaning to the words *desire, hope, motivation,* and *courage.* These are words that you must make your own, in order to color them with the precious energy of joy—joy of feeling and of seeing yourself healing. This joy will progressively help you find the joys of a normal life.

If you succeed in seeing yourself healed and in projecting this certitude into more positive life projects that suit you, all your healing energies will be reinforced and will begin to move more quickly.

So think about it, here and now. Start to think about this fundamental question: What am I going to do with my recovery? Answering with simplicity and lucidity is a shout out to the universe, "Yes, I *want* to get better!" And your unconscious, relieved by your newfound level of maturity, will hear: "Yes, I *can* get better!"

APPENDIX 2

MORE ON
DELTA MEDICINE: FAQS

In this book I have given you a practical synthesis of what my teachers, professional encounters, and life experiences have taught me from the beginning of my medical career to the present. But you may have more questions about my personal background. Here, in the form of a dialogue, I try to respond to some of the more frequently asked questions I receive.

What led you to combine medical approaches that are seemingly so different?

My father was in the military (he was a physician, and passionate about electronics) and my mother was a teacher. To them, life was meant to be approached in a very rigorous, objective, Cartesian way. But during my entire childhood I grew up with my grandmother, a "bonesetter" who treated the inhabitants of her rural area with traditional medicinal plants, using recipes and ritual acts of generosity and healing. These two outlooks on life influenced me profoundly and remained with me as I grew up.

Respecting the wishes of my parents, I began my university coursework by pursuing scientific studies (I myself was passionate about particle physics). But the deep interest I held for the human aspect of science was not fulfilled.

So I resolutely began studies in medicine, followed by neuropsychiatry and neurobiology (in France), and later behavioral neurosciences and nutrition (in the United States, as a graduate student in Boston, where I made valuable contacts with whom I've stayed in touch).

While doing my internship, I had the opportunity (rare at the time) to work in a number of countries, notably in Africa and Asia, where I studied ethnomedicine and the traditional practices of different cultures. Without consciously deciding to, I made the connection between the two main influences of my childhood. These intense experiences soon fostered in me a multidisciplinary and more global concept of medicine, without ever questioning my respect for my teachers and for Western medical science. Looking back, I owe a debt of thanks to a number of my medical teachers, notably Professor San Marco and Professor Marc Alby, for their patience and spirit of openness.

The personal came to join this professional approach when, at the age of twenty-five, I was the victim of a bicycle accident with long-lasting consequences, including intense pains. Unfortunately, the powerful analgesics I was prescribed couldn't be used for long if I wanted to remain lucid on a daily basis. And so, relatively early in my life, I experienced the soothing strengths of breathing exercises and the curative powers of nutrition, notably to limit chronic inflammation. First victory! But following this I developed rheumatoid arthritis (an autoimmune disease) on my traumatized terrain, and the prognosis was terrifying for me. A medical consultant unknowingly predicted that I'd permanently be in a wheelchair within five years. (Somewhat ashamed of being a sick doctor, I had presented my clinical, biological, and radiographic files to him as those of an anonymous patient.) Medicine, "my" medicine, appeared powerless, unable to address my suffering, my illness, and its evolution. Once again, this time with a sense of bitter urgency, I studied nutrition, breathing techniques, and mental imagery ever more attentively. I experimented, refined my practice more and more, and then adopted these measures as part of my daily routine. And I was able to observe their long-lasting positive effects firsthand.

So it was on myself that I first worked and standardized the basis of these techniques, before sharing them with my colleagues, friends, and then with my patients.

I have always kept in mind (and in my heart) the case of a childhood friend diagnosed with advanced-stage bone cancer. She experienced a true remission (judged incredible) after I taught her how to breathe better, eat differently, and relax (along with the treatments she was receiving in the hospital, of course), based, in part, on my ten years of very positive experiences with myself and my patients. I was ecstatic. It was like proof positive of my newfound techniques to promote healing. But six months later, she had a relapse. This deeply hurt and shocked me, and caused me to question myself, and pursue my observations and the quest for long-lasting health with even greater determination.

It was at this time that I started to become very interested in the missing link: emotions. I had been the powerless witness to my friend's ongoing emotional upheaval, which coincided with her illness. I then began to work in the world of neuroscience, turning to Canadian and German schools that place great importance on the symbolic management of emotions. I met other colleagues involved in this field, in France and the United States, who progressively helped me develop two ritualistic protocols of emotional management (outlined in the Delta Psychology chapter of this book). This last therapeutic tool—a tool I developed in a unique collaboration with one of the greatest artists of the human symbolic, Alejandro Jodorowsky—fit in perfectly with the four preceding ones. I regrouped them, standardized them, and organized them so that they would work together in synergy on the five major factors that aid healing (breathing, nutrition, detoxification, management of stress, and emotions) to awaken the healing process.

That is a brief synthesis of my personal and professional background, which has turned out to be the genesis of Delta Medicine, too.

Can holistic techniques, such as breathing, nutrition, or visualization, be enough to heal all illnesses, as some traditional therapeutic schools claim?

Some human beings dedicate their entire life to the practice of physical and spiritual exercises. They give themselves over to it, body and soul, and devote all their time to it. Unquestionably, they have developed some mastery over their bodies, minds, and emotions. But in Western countries, these results are often obtained at a high price—a very intense mental focus, social marginalization, and, sometimes, even alienation from friends and family.

In spite of that, is it possible to prevent all illnesses by devoting your entire life to breathing or meditation practice? The scientific response is complex. I've met yogis, monks, lamas, and sufis who have followed an extreme mind-body discipline and who have avoided all illness. To state with authority that a direct cause-and-effect relationship exists between breathing or meditation practice and illness prevention, a big leap into the unknown must be made, and I cannot make that leap, given the current state of my knowledge. All the same, the life of these mystics, outside the norms of society, is in no way compatible with the human and social criteria that rule our Western lives. Nevertheless, some American universities—Stanford University and the Massachusetts Institute of Technology (MIT), notably—are very seriously and scientifically interested in the almost supernatural powers developed by some Tibetan monks and Hindu yogis. It's clearly proven that they know how to slow their heartbeat at will (or even stop it for several minutes), and can overcome certain infections, control their brain waves, or master their sleep phases. Amazing! But while this is spectacular, I'd like to emphasize that it all lies in opposition to Delta Medicine, because the price to pay for it is often exorbitant on a personal level. Those aren't Delta techniques, but rather mega-techniques, which are marginal and very difficult for most of us to apply, integrate, and master.

This is why I always warn my patients about extreme theories, techniques, and therapies. Attempting to heal yourself by means of just one intense daily practice, whatever it may be (breathing, nutrition, or visualization), poses a great risk of disillusionment (as well as a risk to health). It also undermines your capacity to heal, which dovetails with normalcy and happiness on a daily basis. To my mind, *good health* cannot be defined by the sole criterion of "not being sick." People in good health are those who, if not happy, are at least balanced in their identity, family life, sexuality, relationships, and position in society.

A wholesome environment, simplicity in your lifestyle, and respect for yourself, others, and the planet form the basis of long-term effectiveness of all the Delta techniques. I therefore remain an unconditional advocate for the "extreme center" with regard to all daily choices, including those related to health.

What do you think about the work of well-known doctors, such as O. Carl Simonton and Bernie Siegel, whose work has focused on the mind and emotions in their approach to the fight against cancer?

Nowadays we recognize that the group of holistic doctors from the 1980s, notably Dr. O. Carl Simonton and Dr. Bernie Siegel, were brilliant precursors to contemporary thinking about health and medicine. They have all my respect and admiration. Both of these doctors are serious oncologists. They bring to bear on their work perceptive (and intuitive) medical experience.

During the 1970s and 1980s, they conducted research that led to the beginnings of the field of neuroscience. It took a lot of courage on their part to resolutely move forward, against accepted opinion, on a mental-emotional path that is more and more (and better and better) accepted today (and even in demand at universities and university hospitals). Simonton and then Siegel built the first true bridge between the sick body and the healing mind of the patient. They established credible bases for the first multidisciplinary approach to healing. Neither of them opposed in any way the treatments and procedures of classic medical treatment (they themselves are oncologists, after all).

They saw how to expand the conception of illness, the patient, treatment, healing, and, above all, self-healing. They succeeded at it and today are recognized and respected for their work and their courage as groundbreaking therapists.

This is not necessarily the case for all pioneers working in the field. I'm thinking in particular of someone about whom much has been written, and who incited a wide range of debates (even the suspicion of a medical cult): Dr. Ryke Geerd Hamer, a German doctor who, in spite of all the hoopla surrounding his work, was uniquely intuitive. He thought that all cancer was rooted in an intense emotional shock, and this shock left an imprint within the brain, a sort of active center in the body that became scarred, forming the matrix of all other cancerous tumors. Hoping to come up with scientific proof of his intuitive understanding of cancer at any cost, Dr. Hamer showed the scientific community countless cerebral images (scans and MRIs) with visible traces of these centers. But many of them were distorted by the presence of artifacts. (Artifacts are very common extraneous images that corrupt the cerebral snapshot, a bit like a drop of water on the lens of a camera that makes marks appear on any landscape, resembling a ghostly apparition or a UFO.) This ended up undermining the credibility of his approach. His reputation was equally damaged by some of his disciples, who encouraged their patients to cease all treatments and all medical monitoring (out of respect for the "programmed scarring phase" of the brain!). This attitude was both risky and unconscionable. And it is a therapeutic path that opposes the balanced approach of Simonton and Siegel, and that of Delta Medicine.

Keep in mind that all scientific theory, pushed to the extreme, can get in the way of the patient's healing. The future of medicine belongs to multidisciplinary collaborations, both medical and scientific; to personalized treatments applied to a whole human being and not simply an organic body or symptoms grouped into an illness and treated by various specialists who are not in contact with one another.

It's tempting to think that some of the Delta techniques are more innovative and therefore more effective (or more important) than others. Do you think so?

Here again, citing decades of observations, I can only say that the five tools for health presented in this book are of equal importance with regard to their targeted effectiveness. Their classification (as Tool #1, #2, #3, and so on) is dictated by the order in which I recommend putting them into practice and the ease of comprehension; it is a progressive approach aimed at helping you master the Delta Medicine program. But if I had to classify them according to healing impulse (rather than ease of practice), the order of the five would be:

- First, still, would be Delta Breathing, because of its almost immediate, powerful effect on fear, stress, and the cardiovascular system.
- Next would be Delta Psychology, without any hesitation. It should be started in conjunction with the other tools, and not saved for the end, whenever this is possible (because of the proven success of psychoneuroimmunology in sustaining and reinforcing all our internal mechanisms to fight against cellular abnormalities).
- Then would be Delta Relaxation. It brings to the body new energy and balancing thoughts (very useful on a daily basis and valuable for better managing and supporting chemotherapy and radiation therapy treatments).
- After this would come Delta Detoxification, to help our organs perform their healing functions at 100 percent efficiency (and to ease the shock of prescribed medicines and chemotherapies).
- Finally would be Delta Nutrition, whose daily action is just as powerful (to rebuild a more solid nutritional regimen and digestion). Delta Nutrition involves a true metabolic reprogramming.

This order in no way changes the final result—the awakening of your healing forces. This ideal hierarchy lets us simply reach the heart of mind-body action more rapidly. This proves to be easier when you participate in a complementary medicine group in a hospital (or a specialized clinic like those in the United States, Canada, Germany, England, and Italy). But when a person follows the path of discovering and learning alone, it's better to follow the order listed in this book for maximum effectiveness in three to six weeks.

Most of the Delta Medicine program offers an innovative therapeutic approach, but one that is very structured and understandable. However, the fifth tool, Delta Psychology, may be a bit perplexing. It may hint of New Age mysticism, rather than serious science. How do you respond to that?

The fifth tool for health is very unusual (I'll be more precise and say that it seems very unusual to us and throws us off balance), but it's also highly useful for its originality and overall therapeutic effectiveness within Delta Medicine.

While Delta Psychology is my favorite tool, it's also the tool that has demanded the most research, observation, and truly multidisciplinary collaborations with neurologists, psychiatrists, psychologists, psychoanalysts, ethnomedical doctors, writers, poets, calligraphers, film directors, artists, painters, and singers. Its practical synthesis as a Delta Medicine tool has required years of work.

For many people (both therapists and patients), it will no doubt involve a (re)discovery of that primitive emotional energy so well hidden within the folds of our personality and rendered practically mute by the deafening noise of our modern world. It is a fundamental energy with which we must relearn to interact, but an essential energy to any long-lasting approach to healing and disease prevention.

To use an analogy of our times, you could say that painful, suppressed emotions are to the body what viruses are to computers. It appears as if everything is functioning almost perfectly up until the day when all our life programs are suddenly disrupted. The more you turn on or off the computer, the more the anomalies spread and increase. Eventually, the day comes when you must analyze the situation and reprogram everything. This kind of reprogramming is at the heart of Delta Medicine, and, in particular, of Delta Psychology.

Let us emphasize again that symbolic tools and rituals have played a part in all schools of medicine the world over for more than five thousand years. All our memories and all our emotions form the backdrop or the giant screen for the great film that is our life. If this screen is slightly damaged in one spot, all our life images will bear, or seem to bear, this more or less visible imperfection, depending on the areas of shadow or light on the projected scene. That's why many people often "remain in the shadows" of their own life. Nevertheless, one day we absolutely must stop the film for a few moments and begin to seriously repair our life screen.*

On the other hand, I've clearly emphasized the limits of this tool, which is nothing more than a strategy to reclaim emotional energy. This is essential for us within the context of our will to heal. But all kinds of psychotherapy are there to take over, if necessary (that is, if the damage is too extensive and demands more specialized repair).

Finally, if the acts of health presented in the Delta Psychology program appear surprising or perplexing to an outsider, they do not feel that way to the patient. These symbolic gestures may seem incomprehensible to our sense of reason, but they are very clear words and orders to our unconscious, and that's how they work. I'd be very happy if this tool allowed for a rediscovery of the incredible richness and the incredible therapeutic strength of the energies of the unconscious. I

---

*We can use this colorful comparison to better understand the underlying difference between the world of psychoses and that of neuroses. When a rip on our emotional screen is visible and bothersome, but it doesn't interfere with the projection of the film and the course of our life, this is a neurosis. We're aware of our trouble: it's up to us to find the will to repair our screen. With psychosis, the screen is generally intact but the projection equipment has a technical problem: the life film then becomes weird and incomprehensible without our being able to identify clearly the origin of the problems; in particular there is no precise awareness of these problems (friends and family then spur the decision to consult a therapist). Finally, psychoses and neuroses at times join together in patients called borderline: a large rip on the screen can then be seen, or the projection equipment may fail: it is the mix of the two that, at a minimum, generates personality disorders.

believe that the space for dialogue opened by this new approach to our emotional energies will help tackle questions too often left unanswered (as much for the patient as for the doctor)—those related to the (sometimes strong) emotional distress of our modern world. This is truly one of my deepest wishes springing from the spirit of Delta Psychology.

You present Delta Medicine as a group of tools for health in the service of the healing body, of the body that is its own doctor and calls on all its self-healing energies. But one fundamental question begs to be asked: Are these tools adapted to the infinite variety of ways of breathing, eating, and relaxation; to the infinite variety of thought structures and emotional profiles?

This question may seem abstract, but it leads to an essential reality: Delta Medicine positions itself as a therapeutic tool for the whole body (biological, physical, emotional), but also as a versatile tool, one that is highly adaptable. If you think about it, you'll quickly notice that these techniques affect the five major factors that create (and define) a living human being. Each technique offers enough choices and different points of entry so that all patients can rapidly make it their own. Delta Medicine "offers" the body these techniques, without imposing or asserting them. This adaptability criterion has always guided my choices of which therapy to apply to chronic or degenerative illnesses. The therapy must suit the patient; she must not submit to a therapy that's nearly the same for everyone. It is this adaptability that brings Delta Medicine to life and allows this approach to mesh with what is fully alive in each human being who suffers. It's also a guarantee of reinforced effectiveness, of physical and mental comfort, and of benefits better controlled and therefore more durable.

Can making people breathe differently for a few minutes each day really influence the course of a serious illness?

A different way of breathing, in itself, isn't enough to reverse the course of a serious illness. But breathing more consciously always has a positive effect, even in serious cases of cancer or degenerative diseases. Better control of the breath, in its amplitude and rhythm, can quickly boost the equilibrium of our numerous organs and functions; our thoughts; our stress levels; and enhance our control of our suffering and fears.

This has been observed countless times, and the cause-and-effect relationship has been clearly demonstrated. We know at what point the illness affects our fragile internal equilibrium, and how a regular and controlled breathing practice can contribute to reestablishing that equilibrium. There is nothing simpler than this, even for a child (beginning at age seven, because before that, laughter too quickly prevails over the necessary seriousness for good practice).

Yet many people—patients and doctors alike—still consider breathing a "marginal" or "accessory" practice. This is justified if you refer to the university teachings of the past fifty years. But if you look a little further, you'll notice that breathing techniques have been omnipresent in the traditional medicine and healing rituals of disparate cultures during the past five thousand years. In medicine, we still find some traces of it in obstetrics and gynecology (breathing techniques for labor), in rehabilitation departments (for control of pain), and in some psychiatric departments. But in all cases, these different techniques are only used by motivated treating personnel (midwives, nurses, specialists, physical therapists, psychotherapists), and very rarely by the doctors themselves.

The reason is simple: it's quicker and easier to deliver medication than to teach patients to control their breath and motivate them to regularly practice these exercises. Yet even if we've forgotten, breathing consciously was long ago a sacred act of healing for the Egyptians, the Greeks, the Romans, and the ancient Arab civilizations. It's simple, fast, and easy: these criteria make Delta Breathing of the utmost importance as a therapeutic tool.

Don't all the breathing techniques quickly become tiresome, especially when the patient starts to feel better?

I've integrated Delta Breathing in this form into my medical practice for more than twenty years. And since then, I've never ceased to observe that, once adopted, it remains part of the patient's approach to healing and prevention for life. The large majority of my patients do not practice it grudgingly, but rather they've integrated it into their daily life. The words of one woman of forty, a human relations manager, made a strong impression on me: "It's my peaceful retreat. Wherever I am, during the exercises I truly feel 'at home,' 'inside myself,' in a peaceful place where no one can get at me or harm me. Everything comes into perspective in my head. It's as if my brain also starts breathing." This patient continued to practice Delta Breathing after she recovered from her disease, which was why she had initially come to see me. She never wanted to be destabilized again (that is, to become ill) by nervous and emotional pressure. This Delta space of serenity on demand helped her to keep the pressure and stress from weighing too heavily on the sick side of her health balance.

Discussions on the importance of diet and nutrition are everywhere today. But isn't it too much to ask for the food we choose to eat to intentionally cure us of serious illnesses?

One facet of the medical world regularly rebels against some of the discussions relayed by a media avid for sensationalism—and often justifiably so. Dietary concepts and research findings reported in scientific publications are blithely mixed, watered down, and, even worse, extrapolated to make people see them as miracle cures. In general, those who claim they can heal anything through food base their words on a famous line by Hippocrates, the no less famous father of modern medicine: "Let food be thy medicine." But the message is truncated when conveyed in this way. In fact, Hippocrates expressed this advice in a more nuanced way by asserting: "Let food be thy first medicine." This implies that there are other partners. Of course, reasonable dietary approaches and prevention by good nutrition are extremely effective. But we can't ask for everything. Again, I endorse the idea of a happy medium on a human level as much as a scientific one. The only illnesses susceptible to being "healed" solely by nutritional means are certain kinds of metabolic pathologies very closely linked to food, as is the case in diabetic terrains, gluten allergies, and specific food allergies. For everything else, and notably concerning various kinds of cancer and degenerative diseases, nutritional health is an aid to healing, rather than a cure. It's a precious aid, powerful, and at times even decisive (especially in terms of prevention), but only an aid. Once again, the rules of Delta Nutrition draw their full therapeutic force by supporting all the other tools for health that target cellular, tissue, and then organic equilibrium.

Aren't the discussions related to nutritional trends from different schools of thought, often too disorganized and at times too contradictory for anyone to figure out what the optimal way to eat is?

Nutrition is often presented as a panacea, on the condition that extremely restrictive nutritional directives are followed to the letter for months or even years. To the stress of this constraint is added a kind of mental and social slavery that pushes some people to orthorexia.* The inevitable consequence: The moment will arrive when the constraint is too restrictive, and you return to consuming your usual foods. A relapse is then inevitable, because the previous errors are repeated or even amplified by the rebound effect of frustrations.

Over the course of centuries, humans have shown their extreme adaptability. But we've always remained basically omnivorous, as our tooth structure proves: we have molars to grind and crush, and incisors and canines to cut and rip—all in ideal proportion to ingest and treat all sorts of foods. In every region of the world, the way of eating that dominates (with a few exceptions) is predominantly vegetarian omnivorous. This means that humans nourish themselves mostly with plants (fruits, vegetables, grains, legumes) and, in much smaller proportion, animal sources (meat, fish, dairy products, eggs). This diet, combined with reasonable portions of vegetable oils (cold-pressed), constitutes the way

---

*Orthorexia is the nutritional behavioral disorder that consists of following precise and restrictive dietary advice in an obsessional way, up to the point of making it a rigid lifestyle.

of eating in regions where the highest number of healthy centenarians live.* All the nutritional discussions aimed at breaking this ancestral equilibrium (with the exception of very short lapses of time, for therapeutic purposes, and under medical supervision) are unreasonable and can even prove to be dangerous in the short term.

This is the case for strict vegetarianism, veganism (a dietary approach in which all animal derivatives are forbidden), and raw-food movements, living-food diets, high-protein diets, and fruit diets. Each of our cells has a metabolic memory, and none of them forgets deficiencies or profound imbalances that are imposed on them.

The only situation where I would modify my viewpoint regarding nutrition concerns people for whom restrictive nutritional practices (often linked to vegetarianism or veganism) are integrated into an overall approach at once ecological, humanist, and spiritual. These people succeed at maintaining excellent health because they are generally well-informed and know how to adapt their dietary regimen, as restrictive as it may be, to the essential needs of the body, thanks to specific combinations and complements. I respect their ways. But you must never lose sight of the fact that these are personal choices that involve the person's whole life beyond nutrition. This can in no way replace a medical consultation or treatment protocol, with respect for each of the patients, their family, and their daily life.

We hear so much now about anticancer foods. Why not cover them in your book?

Foods touted as "anticancer" are all over the media. They have been the subject of many successful books. But this very marketable name leads us to believe that these foods are able to directly combat cancer. This seems to me to go beyond the powers of food alone and give false hope to patients. No, you won't heal any kind of cancer or any degenerative illness by filling up on broccoli, kiwi, or papaya. I prefer to adopt a

---

*This is the basis of the famous Mediterranean diet and of the very promising nutritional program from the island of Okinawa.

more prudent and moderate position. Some foods are particularly rich in antioxidants (vitamins and trace elements) and in cell-restoring substances (notably the famous omega-3 fatty acids).

I'd qualify these foods as prohealth, in contrast to the antihealth foods that I talked about in this book (see the purple zone table, page 103). The prohealth foods are beneficial overall to the body, but the act of consuming them in no way influences your nutritional equilibrium. To my mind, they remain essential. The anticancer foods constitute a plus, in the same sense as organic foods. But they only become useful when they're consumed by a body whose metabolic equilibrium has already been reprogrammed by learning the fundamental combinations for health.

What about the macrobiotic diet, whose merits in the treatment of cancer were first promoted in the 1980s?

This kind of diet, founded on the polarity principles of yin and yang that governs Chinese and Japanese medicine, was popularized in Europe during the second half of the twentieth century.* In the 1980s, in a bestselling book, titled *Recalled by Life: The Story of My Recovery from Cancer,* the American physician Dr. Anthony J. Sattilaro recounted how he was cured of cancer by adopting a macrobiotic diet. The strict vegetarian diet is perfectly standardized, with the base food of grains without gluten (rice, principally) and vegetable soups with seaweed and miso (a fermented soy paste, rich in digestive enzymes). After several months of this diet, Dr. Sattilaro saw his symptoms recede dramatically. But after a year of severe dietary restrictions, his Western tastes returned. He dreamed of pasta, bread, and steak. In reality, he had involuntarily committed a great error in judgment: he had only adopted a very small part of the "macrobiotic health structure"—just the diet.

Contrary to what certain media sources stated at the time, this diet

---

*Notably by Georges Oshawa, who wrote several books on the subject, published in Europe; then by his student, Michio Kuchi, in Boston.

is in no way crazy, as long as it's placed within its context. The same is true for the ayurvedic diet from India and the Taoist diet from China. The true macrobiotic diet has five levels, five stages that you must progress through, beginning with a base diet different from the Western dietary regimen (less meat and wheat, more rice and fermented soy). Add to this a strong spiritual dimension (Zen Buddhism) and highly regimented daily practices (massage, meditation, plants). Macrobiotics is an overall lifestyle and not a simple miracle diet.

Nevertheless, you might wonder why Dr. Sattilaro's tumors receded after he adopted a macrobiotic diet. Everything becomes clear if we point out that the last level of macrobiotics, number five, is vegan: the person consumes no animal protein of any kind. The body, deprived of protein, takes protein where it can, but by respecting a specific tissue hierarchy: the cellular masses first, then the muscles, then the digestive organs, the heart, and, finally, the brain (a marvel of nature's good sense). Thus, his body first began by drawing from the tumor, a recent protein mass. That's why this dietary maneuver can be interesting for certain patients, for a limited time (no more than two weeks). But that can't constitute a long-term solution. Of course, at first you may have the impression that the diet directly heals the tumor. But that's not the case. The source of the tumor isn't eradicated and the immune system isn't reinforced. We simply "freeze" the illness at its current point.

The most dangerous trap comes from the fact that, feeling a bit better, patients are tempted to lock themselves away inside this severely deficient and progressively weakening diet. Patients temporarily control an illness that is destroying them with a diet that will, in turn, be just as destructive.

Add to this another danger that, blinded by the sensation of feeling better and unconscious of the fact that it's only transitory, some patients then decide to abandon treatment and classical medical surveillance. And when they finally awaken from this deceptive dream, it's sometimes too late. That's why I firmly warn patients seeking to follow such a route: you must always do it as a complement to the treatment and medical monitoring, and by adopting the entire "ethnotherapeutic" program (body, mind, and spirit, not just nutrition).

Last section on nutrition: Some American and German clinics offer therapeutic fasting programs. Can depriving yourself of food really cure you of an illness?

This question dovetails with the previous one in a couple of ways. Fasting seems to me to be an interesting therapeutic tool, on the express condition that it be correctly controlled and medically supervised. But, here again, this is only a therapeutic tool, in no way an entire therapy. Moreover, this nutritional method can become very dangerous when you "slip." I'm thinking, in particular, of fasts practiced blindly by nonprofessionals and without any medical surveillance. The fast sets off cellular digestion and detoxifying "crises" that can prove beneficial, but at the cost of overworking the organs of elimination—the kidneys, the liver, the gallbladder, and the intestines. Many demands are also placed on the heart and nervous system at the beginning of the program. You must therefore always carefully monitor the state of these organs and their response to the food deprivation. If it turns out that they are the center of a silent weakness (either congenital or acquired), this can awaken and provoke violent, dramatic, detrimental consequences.

I just emphasized that the nervous system is subject to the influence of nutritional contributions. Our digestive system is very rich in nerve cells (neurons), to the point that we often speak of the digestive tract as a "second brain."

Any extreme impact on the digestive system rapidly resonates on the level of the nervous system. A fast can detoxify and recharge an overworked nervous system, when practiced in a clinic and when the faster is cut off from the demands of daily life. But this type of cure can also cause a serious neurosis or a latent mental illness to surface. Fasting is a very specific medical technique, to be handled with many precautions by competent and experienced professionals.

But the total elimination of food,* with the exception of liquids (water, herbal teas, and broth)† can offer certain advantages recognized throughout history. A short-term fast (one to two weeks at most), controlled, with serious biological and psychological monitoring, followed by a progressive and well-timed resumption of food, can effectively give the body a positive biological nudge when it must face a cellular problem. But fasting doesn't cure anything. It only reprograms certain facets of the body's internal equilibrium, which patients must take control of (consciously and seriously) after the end of the fast if they want to avoid an even more severe return of the original problems.

What is the place of detoxification in the overall Delta Medicine regimen?

All the Delta techniques call on nonchemical strategies but are not to be classified among medicines called natural or alternative, as I already emphasized. These are personalized therapeutic programs designed to awaken our healing forces. When I suggest that readers learn to breathe better and balance their diet before detoxifying the body, this is not without reason: the effects of a detoxification cure are very transitory if you are not careful to first modify your (bad) daily habits. If you don't do this, the reintoxication and the recontamination of the body will be very rapid and all your efforts will have been in vain.

While we are on the subject, I'd like to add a practical remark that I consider very important regarding medicinal plants. In phytotherapy books, the recommended infusion times are very long (ten minutes on average), while in the Delta Detox program, I suggest infusing for only two or three minutes. In fact, the infusion time depends on the active ingredients that you want to extract from the plant and therefore on the kind of action you wish to obtain. Long infusions (and

---

*This deprivation can also be partial (reduced to just one food consumed plain), as in the case of monodiets.

†Beware: certain extreme fasts also advocate the elimination of liquids for two or three days. This can result in irreversible damage to the kidneys.

decoctions)* are useful when you want to absorb the healing properties of a therapeutic plant for several days to address an acute problem. But the body doesn't tolerate this strong concentration of active ingredients over the long term, and herbal teas that are too concentrated end up provoking intestinal problems (bloating, colitis, or diarrhea). In this book, I suggest drinking herbal teas that can be consumed regularly over a very long period, without the least risk of unpleasant side effects. Within this context, detox mixtures infused for two or three minutes are not only sufficient to be effective, but extremely well tolerated by the body in the long term.

What might be the place of alternative modalities like homeopathy, phytotherapy, or acupuncture in the treatment of cancers?

These therapeutic treatments may be tolerated in particular private practices, but they aren't always well accepted by the scientific community. Personally, I don't know if Professor Jacques Benvéniste's famous studies on water memory in the 1990s were illusory or revolutionary, but at the same time, these studies were taken up again more recently by Professor Luc Montagnier, winner of the Nobel Prize in medicine in 2008. I don't know if the famous energy meridians that acupuncturists work on constitute a biological reality or a simple symbolic image offered by Chinese medicine, which is five thousand years old. I'm unaware of whether there exist today on our planet medicinal plants capable of curing or slowing the progress of cellular problems; that is, true anticancer plants.

What I do know, on the other hand, is that these therapeutic approaches, delivered by professionals, beyond the debates and sterile polemics, can often provide valuable mind-body help to patients. In fact, doctors trained in these kinds of practices generally devote more time to listening to their patients, and their questionnaires leave more space

---

Decoction refers to the action of infusing the plant in boiling water and letting it boil from three to thirty minutes, depending on the part of the plant being used. Decoctions are most often made from roots.

for details about a patient's mental and emotional life. The therapeutic tools at their disposal can promote better tolerance (psychological and physical) of other treatments, and help stimulate a person's healing and self-healing forces.

Yet, these medical approaches must not and cannot be a substitute for allopathic treatments and protocols. Steer clear of therapists—doctors or not—who from the very first consultation advise you to have complete confidence in them and abandon allopathic treatments just like that. And don't forget that the only person in whom you can have total and complete confidence is yourself. But a "you" invigorated with good sense, a healthy conscience, the right surroundings, and the motivation to share the journey of healing with your medical team. Homeopathy, acupuncture, phytotherapy, trace element therapy, and ayurvedic medicine only have a real place (which they must continue to refine and affirm) at the heart of a multidisciplinary approach to illness.

One word on osteopathy and chiropractic: Are these approaches reserved for backaches, or are they really useful as an adjunct in the treatment of various kinds of cancer?

My opinion is both nuanced and moderate. I've had the chance to be associated with the best in this discipline, at the highest levels of competitive sports (for joint and muscle troubles). But then I met up again with these same therapists at the bedside of many gravely ill patients.

As they explain it themselves, when you reestablish equilibrium in the structures, muscles, tendons, and fascia, that influences the equilibrium of the whole body. In the body, everything's connected. Take the example of the thoracic vertebrae: each vertebra that is "freed," each paravertebral muscle that is "despasmed," strengthens all the nervous connections of the target organs (liver, spleen, pancreas, kidneys, and digestive tract). It's the same for the cervical vertebrae, whose "liberation" sends rebalancing impulses to the thymus, the thyroid, and all the lymphatic ganglia of this area.

My personal conclusion on a practical level: Choosing with (great) care, I always recommend one or two checkup visits with an osteopath or chiropractor—regardless of whether or not the patient has a backache. In the same spirit I recommend that my patients make one or two visits to their dentist to check old fillings, bimetallism,* decay, or granuloma, which is silent but very toxic on cellular and cardiac levels within a few years.

Do traditional medicines have a place in the treatment of cellular problems and degenerative illnesses?

When I talk about ethnomedicine, keep in mind that I am excluding unscrupulous charlatans—they're easy to spot these days with a bit of good sense and thanks to networks of recognized associations of competent therapists found on the Internet. The true kinds of ethnomedicine are practiced by therapists seriously trained in these demanding disciplines. These therapists draw from an ancient tradition (sometimes more than five thousand years old) and offer a large palette of complementary gestures that act together in synergy: nutritional advice, draining techniques, massages, relaxation or meditation techniques, and/or medicinal plant cocktails. As Westerners, we must only get involved in all good conscience, with curiosity, but, above all, with good sense. You must understand what you're undergoing and what you're doing. Keep in mind your Western points of reference, of seriousness and safety, while opening yourself to the holistic spirit and to a larger vision of the overall body.

Let's not forget that more than half the world's population does not have access to modern medical techniques, and these people heal themselves only with these local traditional medicines. These populations

---

*This is the presence of different metals to fill teeth (silver and gold, silver and iron, or even gold and iron). Bimetalism leads to the appearance of an electrical current and progressive ionization of the saliva, which affects the digestion, the blood quality, and the production of free radicals. Serious problems can result from this in both the short term and the long term.

haven't all been decimated by illness—far from it. Traditional healers have at their disposal effective plant-based herbal remedies (macerations, decoctions, powders of mixed dried plants). And almost 80 percent of the molecules on which our modern drugs are based have been copied from the active ingredients in plants. China, for example, has a vast traditional pharmacopoeia and has just opened its worldwide pharmaceutical market within the past few decades.

That hasn't stopped people from surviving numerous epidemics, century after century.

In recalling that, I in no way minimize Western medicine's superb discoveries, which have helped save countless lives. But there is an inescapable biological law: the longer a medicinal molecule is active, the more it provokes side effects. It is therefore worthwhile to choose therapeutic tools that will be used according to the urgency of the illness. Facing a serious motor vehicle accident, the IVs, anesthesia, painkillers, cerebral anti-inflammatory drugs, and surgeries are irreplaceable. But that in no way means we should neglect additional strategies that help accelerate convalescence. Bravo for the powerful antibiotics that help curb bacterial infections! But let's not forget the indispensable renewal of intestinal flora. Facing a tumorous cancer, chemotherapy, radiation therapy, and surgery remain remarkably valuable. But following a regimen of these techniques doesn't necessarily imply that you must renounce the long-lasting benefits that other medical techniques of healing can bring.

Viral infections are a slightly different story. A virus is not, strictly speaking, a living organism, but a dead protein coding. It must colonize our cells to become living, which makes it terribly destructive. Antibiotic molecules have no effectiveness on these viruses, which nestle inside our own cells, protected. It's a primary health problem to which medicine has not been able to deliver an effective response to date. Once again, it is here that traditional medicines have a role to play, to reinforce the terrain and stimulate our own immune defenses.

I must emphasize that the current worldwide problem presented by viruses is particularly severe, beyond media clichés and catastrophic scenarios of large pandemics. These same viruses are triggering factors, aggravating or associated with certain kinds of cancer and autoimmune diseases.

This problem is all the more serious because viruses mutate very rapidly. All they need to do this is to reorganize a few coding molecules. Reinforcing our own defenses thus seems like the best solution for the moment when we're facing unpredictable and unstable cellular enemies. To succeed at this, the weapons at our disposal are a healthy diet, detoxification, correct breathing, and management of stress and emotions. We always come back to that: a biological, nervous, and emotional terrain that is stronger will allow us to live with viruses without getting sick.

Claude Bernard's sentence returns like a leitmotif: the virus is nothing—it's the terrain that makes the difference.

A more marginal question that you hear a lot about at the moment: What are the diagnostic theories and therapeutic applications of symbolic psychological approaches and biological decoding all about?

This very trendy niche seduces many patients with its magical diagnostics. The great French leaders of this current are Dr. Salomon Sellam and Dr. Claude Sabbah.

In summary, each organ affected by an illness carries within it a signature, symbolically linked to a particular emotion. Some simple examples: The liver refers to suppressed anger, the throat to something unpleasant that remains in the way, the kidneys to an attack on our vital territory, skin to a notion of an emotional stain, and so on. There are many books on the topic; don't hesitate to consult them to go beyond this brief summary.

Two quite parallel worlds confront each other with regard to this diagnostic approach. On the one hand, universities cry charlatanism and abuse of trust. On the other hand, these therapists (doctors or not) cry sabotage, obscurantism, and bad faith. Strangely, I believe that the two parties could both be partially right, but each in their own way.

I hesitated a long time before voicing my opinion on these particular concepts. But after several years, two things convinced me to do so: first, the growing presence of these diagnostic approaches in the milieu of those who are seriously ill; and second, the rereading of some of Carl Gustav Jung's work (one of the major precursors of modern symbolic thinking). This is why I give you this key passage, accompanied by the commentary of Jung himself who, unbeknownst to him, gives a revealing response to the debate about biological decoding that now animates the medical world.

Jung obviously didn't know and thus didn't directly apply this technique of mind-body decoding, but he handled the symbolic with amazing dexterity. He was a therapist without equal. For example, in 1933 Jung had to interpret the following dream at the request of a patient and his doctor.

> Near me, someone was asking questions about how to lubricate a machine. Someone else suggested that milk would be the best lubricant. Apparently, I thought that it would be better to use liquid mud. Then a pond was emptied and in the sludge were two animals— extinct species. One was a minuscule mastodon, the other, I don't remember anymore.

Jung then diagnosed in an incredibly precise way (and magical, for the layperson as much for the doctor) cerebrospinal fluid retention. He based his interpretation on the fact that one of the "muddy" liquids of the body is called *pituita* in Latin, and that the word *mastodon* is derived from two Greek words meaning "mammal" and "tooth." From there he deduced that the image of the mastodon corresponded to the corpus mamillare, structures shaped like breasts situated under the third ventricle, the pond of cerebrospinal fluid at the base of the brain.

If these weren't the words of one of the most reputable psychoanalysts in the world, it would at best bring a smile to the face of a layman, and at worst elicit a cry of fraud from a therapist.

Pressed by his colleagues at the time to explain himself, and questioned on the way in which he had arrived at such a conclusion, Jung simply responded:

Why does it seem obvious to me that this dream reveals an organic symptom? If I explained it to you, you'd accuse me of the most terrible obscurantism. When I talk about archetypes, those among you who are informed understand me, but those who aren't, think: "This guy is completely crazy. He's talking about mastodons and their differences with snakes and horses." I'd have to give you a four-semester course on the symbolic before you could appreciate what I said.

And Jung thus gives the clearest and most elegant response concerning all the new diagnostic and healing techniques, all that official science considers borderline, all that is considered alternative therapeutics.

You can only communicate, teach, and be socially and scientifically credible with the same life referents, whether intellectual or cultural. Doctors who go back to the sources of ethnomedicine respect them, understand them, and apply them much better than if they had learned it in books. Because at the source, human energy, tradition, and the symbolic mix harmoniously.

Jung thus "seemed" to diagnose complex pathologies in a "miraculous" way, based on the symbolic interpretation of dreams. His approach was totally scientific, ethical, and honest, on the basis of his own knowledge, his own (immense) cultural understanding, and his own (unique) sensitivity. Yet his diagnostic technique remains difficult to teach in universities, because our standard cultural references are insufficient. The interested doctors would have to agree to develop their "being" (emotions) more than their "having" (mental knowledge).

Are we ready for that? Yes, I sincerely think that the current scientific and medical generation is open to—even eagerly anticipating—these new human impulses.

But we must not forget that Jung, while curious and very cultivated, was also respectful of the biological medicine of his time and, in the end, prudent, moderate, and patient.

If therapists convinced by symbolic psychology could bring together these "few" fine qualities, as Jung did, then a future in which to refine their motivating intuition would certainly await us.

In conclusion, this diagnostic approach still remains very marginal, and is to be approached with caution. Its pertinence seems to be dependent on the competence and mental and psychological maturity of the therapist, as well as her certification (in the sense of associated medical knowledge). There also exists the possibility of encountering incompetent practitioners or charlatans advocating for this stylish ideological movement. Unfortunately, they can, in an attractive and theatrical way, present the form of this technique without mastering the essence; that is, the substance. Once again, the same warning applies: choose doctors or psychologists having, beyond the competencies required of their discipline, an additional, indispensable competency—the ethics associated with the capacity to know their limits. And, once again, refuse any unofficial modification of your medical protocol in progress, without direct and supported collaboration from your team of doctors and nurses.

It seems a little surprising that you would cover numerous degenerative diseases and lifestyle diseases without once mentioning AIDS (acquired immune deficiency syndrome). Why?

My position is very clear: it's a question of respect. Respect for the medical structures in place. Respect for all the national and international associations that have done extraordinary work in response to the AIDS epidemic over the past twenty years. These patient associations, coordinated by patients themselves, have understood before anyone else the importance of the terrain, whether biological, nutritional, mental, or emotional. The multidisciplinary therapeutic approaches and the holistic coordination of the most diverse human competencies have been the rule since the beginning of this fight. It's a fight that inspires strong emotions—even more so respect and humility—in all doctors and researchers.

"Soliciting," even involuntarily, seems anathema to me. That's why I make no allusion to AIDS in this book. By talking about it here, in the appendix, in the form of a direct dialogue, I can let myself respond with a resounding *Yes!*

Yes, I think Delta Medicine's tools for health can accompany AIDS patients on the path to well-being, in the long term.

Yes, I think the tools are useful on a daily basis to support the quality of life and the hope of a remission, of a long-lasting "viral silence." But it is up to the associations* or individuals who come across my book to decide whether or not to adopt Delta Medicine's health strategies. Their intuitions will be stronger than my convictions.

---

*These associations also promote the immune health of patients by the sheer force and quality of their human contacts and the mission they share with their members.

APPENDIX 3

ANNOTATED BIBLIOGRAPHY

Today there are hundreds of serious publications and thousands of pertinent bibliographic references that integrate scientific concepts targeting the five tools for health covered in this book.

In three decades, I've had access to more than a thousand studies and books, both French and international, that have caught my attention: more than half of them can still be found in my library, and I page through them from time to time, whenever questions arise. More often than not, the questions need to be answered in the face of new cases, new health challenges.

Nevertheless, as I started writing this before a wall of books, I looked back on my professional and personal background: What were the key moments in my life, and what remarkable readings were connected to them? In thirty years, five key moments have allowed me to evolve (and, at times, progress) in my medical practice, and fifteen or more books were associated with them.

I've listed them in the pages that follow, sometimes with personal annotations and sometimes with suggested books that could accompany them (or are of the same ideological persuasion).

Most of the books are equally suitable for patients or those seeking to prevent illness as well as scientists and health professionals. I have indicated those books that are primarily geared toward one or the other.

Happy reading! I hope that once or twice you'll be surprised as much as I was.

HOLISTIC ONCOLOGY AND
AUTOIMMUNE AND DEGENERATIVE DISEASES

Schwartz, Laurent. *Cancer: A Dysmethylation Syndrome.* Montrouge, France: John Libbey Eurotext, 2005.

————. *Cancer: Between Glycolysis and Physical Constraint.* Berlin/New York: Springer, 2004.

Two superb works of scientific competence and sincerity, by a colleague who is abrasive but lucid, passionate, and riveting. His ideas are right on point. Schwartz probes new fields of research, taking a different approach from that of Delta Medicine, but he offers cancer patients hope, based on solid research. These technical tomes are aimed at professionals, but motivated patients may also find them accessible.

Servan-Schreiber, David, and Robert Laffont. *Anticancer: A New Way of Life.* New York: Viking, 2009.

A man, a doctor, and a big name. But also a man of courage: Servan-Schreiber won his bet and recovered from cancer! A reference work that has made enough of an impression on the general public and the media so that the word *cancer* will never again be pronounced in a powerless tone by patients, doctors, or those in the news media.

Siegel, Bernie S. *Love, Medicine, and Miracles.* New York: Harper & Row, 1986.

Written more than twenty-five years ago by a doctor who is a cancer specialist, this book describes a unique approach, a way of thinking and intuition that is out of the ordinary, an opening and expansion of O. Carl Simonton's thinking (see p. 232), and a humanity without limits, which is in itself therapeutic. A book of great sensitivity and an excellent work for the revival of holistic thinking in oncology. Everyone should read it: patients, those who are well, and doctors and therapists from all schools of thought.

Matthews-Simonton, Stephanie. *The Healing Family*. New York: Bantam, 1984.

Simonton, O. Carl, Stephanie Matthews-Simonton, and James L. Creighton. *Getting Well Again*. Los Angeles: J. P. Tarcher, 1978.

Simonton, O. Carl, and Reid Henson. *The Healing Journey*. New York: Bantam, 1992.

These are three reference books on the Simonton method, one of the largest movements to revive mind-body medicine, which was launched in the second half of the twentieth century. A nice mastery of guided mental imagery at the service of a superb therapist. A basis of reflection and research during my first stay in the United States in the 1980s. A unique influence on thousands of new mind-body–school doctors in countries throughout the world.

THERAPEUTIC NUTRITION AND DIETARY HEALTH PROGRAMS

Campbell, T. Colin, and Thomas M. Campbell. *The China Study: The Most Comprehensive Study of Nutrition Ever Conducted and the Startling Implications for Diet, Weight Loss, and Long-Term Health.* Dallas: BenBella Books, 2006.

The most extensive international study to date on nutrition. Reflections and directions to consider in spite of the conclusions, which I find too committed to one viewpoint.

Vasey, Christopher. *The Acid–Alkaline Diet for Optimum Health: Restore Your Health by Creating pH Balance in Your Diet.* Rochester, Vt.: Healing Arts Press, 2006.

Naturopath Christopher Vasey shows how a simple change in diet to restore your acid–alkaline balance can result in vast improvements in health.

Willcox, Bradley J., Craig Willcox, and Makoto Suzuki. *The Okinawa Program*. New York: Three Rivers Press, 2001.

Authored by a team of internationally renowned experts, this book is based on the twenty-five-year Okinawa Centenarian Study, a Japanese Ministry of Health–sponsored study. This book reveals the diet, exercise, and lifestyle practices that make the Okinawans the healthiest and longest-lived population in the world.

PHYTOTHERAPY

There are a dozen serious books on this topic. All are good for familiarizing yourself with plants. But be careful: phytotherapy and aromatherapy (therapy with essential oils) are not mild medicines, even if they're natural and holistic. Plants are very powerful healing agents and are therefore sometimes highly toxic. Always seek advice about the doses, the dosage form, and the way the plants are administered.

Also be careful because any plants coming from Asia, Africa, or South America must not be ordered on the Internet—numerous counterfeits exist and are sometimes toxic. Medical advice is always suggested. For all mixtures of plants suggested in these books, you should speak with a knowledgeable pharmacist or a registered herbalist (this is ideal).

Hoffmann, David. *Medical Herbalism: The Science and Practice of Herbal Medicine*. Rochester, Vt.: Healing Arts Press, 2003.

Geared toward the professional, this is a foundational textbook on the scientific principles of therapeutic herbalism and their application in medicine.

Schnaubelt, Kurt. *The Healing Intelligence of Essential Oils: The Science of Advanced Aromatherapy*. Rochester, Vt.: Healing Arts Press, 2011.

Written by the founder and scientific director of the Pacific Institute of Aromatherapy in San Francisco, this book explores science's new biological understanding of essential oils for improved immunity and treatment of degenerative diseases.

Treben, Maria. *Health through God's Pharmacy: Advice and Proven Cures with Medicinal Herbs.* Steyr, Austria: Ennsthaler Publishing, 2009.

For decades now, the bestselling book in Europe on phytotherapy, written for the general public. Features excellent, old-fashioned remedies and showcases the editor's wonderful knowledge of the best known and most widely used nontoxic plants in the countryside. But too much liberty is taken with the tone of the book, which often renders the research facilities cited not credible. The book is worth reading for its practical applications; the magical aspect is definitely forgettable.

Valnet, Jean. *The Practice of Aromatherapy: A Classic Compendium of Plant Medicines and Their Healing Properties.* Rochester, Vt.: Healing Arts Press, 1990.

A colleague of mine, who has devoted his life to phytotherapy, and who has earned worldwide renown in his field. This book covers 40 essences in detail, providing scientific explanations for how they work and detailed instructions for internal and external use of the plants.

Winston, David, and Steven Maimes. *Adaptogens: Herbs for Strength, Stamina, and Stress Relief.* Rochester, Vt.: Healing Arts Press, 2007.

The definitive guide to adaptogenic herbs, formerly known as "tonics," that counter the effects of age and stress on the body.

MIND-BODY MEDICINE
AND TAKING CONTROL OF ILLNESS

Benson, Herbert, and William Proctor. *Relaxation Revolution: Enhancing Your Personal Health through the Science and Genetics of Mind Body Healing.* New York: Scribner, 2010.

Benson, Herbert, and Ellen M. Stuart. *The Wellness Book: The Comprehensive Guide to Maintaining Health and Treating Stress-Related Illness.* New York: Fireside, 1992

Benson, of Harvard Medical School, has dedicated his life to proving that meditative responses tangibly improve physical health, reduce illness, and encourage a healthy immune response. He utilizes conventional research methods and rigorously tests a variety of illnesses.

Borysenko, Joan. *Minding the Body, Mending the Mind.* Cambridge, Mass.: Da Capo Press, 2007.
Based on Dr. Borysenko's groundbreaking work at the Mind/Body Clinic in Boston, this book is a classic in the field. The clinic's dramatic success with thousands of patients—with conditions ranging from allergies to cancer—offers vivid proof of the effectiveness of the mind-body approach to health.

Cousins, Norman. *Anatomy of an Illness as Perceived by the Patient.* New York: W. W. Norton and Co., Inc., 1979.
A huge classic of American literature, written by a political journalist who was a master of practical intuition, good sense, and a will to live in good health. Geared toward laypeople rather than health professionals.

Hirshberg, Caryle, and Marc Ian Barasch. *Remarkable Recovery.* New York: Riverhead Books, 1996.
Jaffe, Dennis T. *Healing from Within.* New York: Alfred A. Knopf, 1980.
Weil, Andrew. *Spontaneous Healing.* New York: Alfred A. Knopf, 1995.
Three great classics from the American multidisciplinary (holistic) therapeutic tradition. Dynamic writing, well-documented books, easy and motivating reads, and high-quality, practical advice. However, some passages need to be updated, given the current context of mind-body medicine practiced in hospitals. These works will appeal primarily to laypeople rather than health professionals.

Janssen, Thierry. *The Solution Lies Within: Towards a New Medicine of Body and Mind.* London: Free Association Books, 2010.
A medical doctor, a surgeon, and a psychotherapist, the author offers

a very comprehensive reflection on the numerous facets of healing. The psychosomatic route and traditional medicine play leading roles here.

Siebert, Al. *The Survivor Personality*. New York: Perigee Trade, 2010.
Excerpt from the convention of the Western Psychology Association (April 1983).

PSYCHOSOMATIC TRAINING, BREATHING, RELAXATION, AND GUIDED MENTAL IMAGERY

Here we find the great therapeutic movements of the twentieth century, whose effectiveness has been largely demonstrated and well standardized: those of Dr. Johannes Heinrich Schultz, Dr. O. Carl Simonton, Professor Julian de Ajuriaguerra, Sapir, and Ericksonian hypnosis. The most famous, practical, and approachable remains that of Dr. Schultz (the renowned autogenic training). **Most of the specific titles I would recommend are not currently available in English. However, the resourceful reader can easily find more information about these techniques online or in your local bookshop.** In the past decade, there has been renewed interest in autogenic training among the general public, who are increasingly seeking out natural, holistic solutions in response to the mounting and intolerable pressures from professional and personal stress.

These techniques mobilize the body through a special series of exercises, with the goal of positively influencing the equilibrium and resources of the entire nervous system. Nevertheless, three very simple and very effective exercises are too often forgotten: fast walking (while swinging the arms fully), dancing, and singing. Also worth exploring are schools that integrate Western methods of body expression (Feldenkrais, art therapy, Pilates) with the Eastern modalities (different styles of yoga, conscious walking). Finally, there are multiple exercises for the breath or the more modern neurolinguistic programming. There are many books, both practical and competent on all of these methods, and they can be selected according to the physical path to relaxation that seems best for you.

SELF-ANALYSIS AND OPENING
THE MIND TO CONSCIOUSNESS

This last part of the bibliography is the most specific. It is to encourage the patient—or anyone in good health who wants to remain so—to begin or complete self-analysis. It is what we have called an aware approach.

This is a very personal domain that we will cover from a strictly nonreligious point of view (related to the medical mindset and out of respect for the patient). Experience shows that work on the self and a desire to open up our mind can be a great source of support during a serious or chronic illness.

All these titles are accessible (but never simplistic) and offer practical approaches and routes to reflection. Without claiming to change lives, these books can positively influence them. Sometimes this can represent a big step, even a decisive step.

Dass, Ram. *Still Here: Embracing Aging, Changing, and Dying.* New York: Riverhead Books, 2001.
Lovely thoughts on spirituality and daily wisdom by way of autobiographical anecdotes, full of humor and an incredible level of maturity. A true breath of serenity.

Desjardins, Arnaud. *Toward the Fullness of Life: The Fullness of Love.* Prescott, Ariz.: Hohm Press, 1995.
———. *The Jump Into Life: Moving Beyond Fear.* Prescott, Ariz.: Hohm Press, 1994.
Desjardins is one of the most spiritually mature authors of the twentieth century. These books are more relevant than ever now, at the beginning of the third millennium, when emotional confusion reigns. To be read outside of any belief system. Clear, practical writing of the highest quality, lovely lines of thought, and personal solutions. Arnaud Desjardins doesn't give rigid advice and he doesn't attempt to define wisdom; he simply

radiates it and passes it on. He is in full possession of this authority and has devoted his whole life to sharing his wisdom with us.

Hanh, Thich Nhat. *Breathe You Are Alive: The Sutra on the Full Awareness of Breathing.* Berkeley, Calif.: Parallax Press, 2008.
———. *Peace Is Every Breath: A Practice for Our Busy Lives.* New York: HarperOne, 2011.
———. *Peace Is Every Step: The Path of Mindfulness in Everyday Life.* New York: Bantam, 1992.
———. *Transformation and Healing: Sutra on the Four Establishments of Mindfulness.* Berkeley, Calif.: Parallax Press, 1990.
Profound, incredibly human writings from a Vietnamese monk living in France, with an understanding of the Western consciousness and way of thinking. Practical, very credible exercises from recent developments in the neurosciences.

Jodorowsky, Alejandro. *Psychomagic: The Transformative Power of Shamanic Psychotherapy.* Rochester, Vt.: Inner Traditions, 2010.
———. *The Spiritual Journey of Alejandro Jodorowsky.* Rochester, Vt.: Park Street Press, 2008.
Must-read books for anyone who wants to approach spirituality with serious intention without taking himself too seriously. The author has developed his incredible talent as a holistic storyteller, touching the deepest recesses of the human soul. He also discusses the power that symbols and symbolic gestures have over our unconscious. His discourse is linked to the essence of Delta Medicine's fifth tool (Delta Psychology).

Jung, Carl Gustav. *The Basic Writings of C. G. Jung.* Edited by Violet Staub de Laszlo. New York: Modern Library, 1993.
———. *Modern Man in Search of a Soul.* First published in 1933. Boston: Harcourt Harvest, 1955.
———. *The Undiscovered Self: With Symbols and the Interpretation of Dreams.* Translated by R. F. C. Hull. New York: Mentor, 1958.

The genius and therapeutic intuition of a great doctor and a great thinker of the twentieth century. Any commentary is superfluous. These challenging works are recommended primarily for scientists and health professionals. You must simply read it and reread it for yourself, and don't lose the wish to learn more.

Long, Barry. *Only Fear Dies*. Los Angeles: Barry Long Books, 1996.

A direct reflection on our fundamental fears, without any concessions. These resurfacing fears can weigh heavily on our personal trials and illnesses. Practical, credible solutions, because they all come from the courage of a lived experience, the work of one whole life. Words that enliven us to search for our own bits of courage.

I'm sure some excellent books are missing from this (nonexhaustive) list. I have not yet had the pleasure of reading them all, and beg the pardon of their authors. I'm quite sure to have missed as many good ones as I've cited. But with the miracle of the Internet you can of course connect to the sites of major online bookstores and search by themes or authors for any and all titles missing from this bibliographic appendix.

Be both curious and clear-sighted. Only believe what you can verify, always with the approval of—in collaboration with—the medical team treating you. Above all, believe in what is good for you, physically and mentally, and claim it for yourself!

Remember that each day everything is possible. But don't forget that a part of everything depends on you. And only you.

It depends on your motivation, your involvement, and your regular practice of the tools for health. Never again play games with yourself: think, and act freely and positively.

Be fully alive, and do everything you can to stay that way!

APPENDIX 4

THE CHALLENGE OF NEUROSCIENCES

This short recap of the latest research in neuroscience is essentially meant to emphasize one point still little recognized by the general public, and sometimes the medical world itself, with regard to the current state of affairs in science—the spectacular evolution of several multidisciplinary programs of prevention and therapeutic intervention in the past decade. Just as spectacular are the advances in neuroscience, in particular, and in mind-body medicine in general (with the recognition, application, and teaching of psychoneuroimmunology in the United States and Canada and, since 2005, in many European university hospitals in Germany, Belgium, the United Kingdom).

One confirmed observation in France by Robert Dantzer, director of a research group in Bordeaux, which specializes in stress and the physiopathology of cellular communication:

> The rapid evolution of knowledge about interactions between the nervous system and the immune system is exemplary from the psychosomatic point of view, because it concerns a domain where the possible relationship between mental factors and the pathology have been the source of many controversies, without there being the smallest fact to argue in one direction or the other. The situation has changed completely over the last eight years. We are now capable of

explaining how a mental state can have an effect on the functioning of the immune system and how illness can affect the mental system.

This from his excellent book, *L'Illusion psychosomatique (The Psychosomatic Illusion)*, published by Odile Jacob in 2001.

What follows regroups the bibliographic summaries of some discoveries and lines of research whose conclusions are at the root of the Delta Medicine program (along with personal experience and numerous exchanges with colleagues). These bibliographic trails don't explain everything—far from it. But they allow for a positive, reasonable, and ethical integration of the tools of Delta Medicine in all the classic medical therapeutic protocols.

If you discover these new therapeutic methods all at once and this upends your former certainties, resist the temptation to search for a shortcut to calm your frustrations. Resist the reflex of the pat answer: "Of course, the author only presents what backs up his personal theses. He tells us this or that as a 'fact,' but I've 'seen' another study saying exactly the opposite. So what does it matter?" Resist this "shut-down reflex" of the mind and take the time to really study and understand what is shown and suggested, the product of attentive readings of (and research into) all the scientific arguments developed in these publications.

I must remind both colleagues and patients that studies targeting the biological sites of action and feedback loops of simple aspirin (salicylic acid) are still incomplete, and certainly contradictory. We find the same arguments alive and well (and often exacerbated by economic stakeholders, for different classes of anti-inflammatories, antimigraine drugs, hypotensives, cholesterol-lowering drugs, vaccinations, and, of course, for all classes of anticancer medications (many protocols returning to molecules discovered a decade ago, abandoned, and then updated for lack of anything better).

So I think that it's best to maintain a pronounced taste for the happy medium: all these questions still exist, but they in no way stop us from treating cancerous and degenerative illnesses better and better.

I support without reservation the positive realism of our colleague Professor Anne Ancelin-Schützenberger when she states, "The fear of cancer is more harmful than the cancer itself. These days cancer is cured, and cured often. People die less from cancer than from heart attacks or accidents."

I also support without reservation the scientists, researchers, and hospital workers who in all good conscience bet on the "reasonable" fact that several studies, led by different teams and coming to the same conclusions, can contain an element of truth that can be used in therapeutics with respect for the patient.

I maintain that it's reasonable to try regrouping all that's naturally positive for human beings, sometimes without having fully mastered all the mechanisms of the actions or biophysiological interactions. (I refer here to natural health techniques related to physical or mental health training programs. Chemical therapies and various medications must be evaluated with much greater scrutiny, targeting as precisely as possible the toxic risks and the effects specifically toxic for pregnant women and the fetus.)

The tools for health presented in the Delta Medicine program have technically delivered proof of their positive impacts on the overall state of health of many patients and on that of the patients' biological terrain. Neurophysiological schemas that are even more comprehensive will be created, step by step, in the coming decades.

For now we must keep an open mind, encourage patient motivation to become part of our practice, and see as often as possible a magnificent synergy of healing aid at work: the medicine made by humans at the service of the body's own medicine.

Here, to complete this bibliography, is a selection of recent studies targeting the medical techniques grouped under the generic title of "mind-body medicine." These studies come directly from the most recent advances in neuroscience and the mind-body approach emphasized throughout this book.

The scientific magazine *Science et Vie* (Science and Life)—serious, ethical, and well documented—echoes this wonderful synthesis very clearly with this article title from its November 2004 issue: "Psychomedicines: When the Mind Saves the Body—The Challenge of Neurosciences."

The new therapeutic momentum that I hoped to offer as a daily practice in this book on Delta Medicine cannot be summarized better than it is in the introduction by the assistant editor of *Science et Vie,* Philippe Chambon.

> The powers of the mind on the body are irrefutable: this is the verdict from the surprising experiments that demonstrate that not only does the mind act on the body, but it succeeds in healing it! . . . The stakes are scientific as well as medical. Doctors are conducting these experiments. And for good reason: that the mind acts on the body is a fantastic therapeutic lead. And this ought to evolve mentalities. Medicine and psychology can finally stop looking askance at one another. Not that the body guard would yield to the spirit protector on the question of scientific rigor. Quite the contrary. But these two enemies, confronted with the limits of their art, are now forced to ally their forces and reason in order to take on the responsibility of human suffering, beyond prejudices and preconceptions.

Molecular medicine and mind-body medicine are therefore forced to ally their therapeutic forces. This new synergy is one of the foundations of the practical program of Delta Medicine.

The titles of the major experiments cited in this article do not constitute the synthesis of perfect biological schemas but of irrefutable, practical, and very promising ways to promote healing.

Psychological Support Stimulates Immune Defenses

Study led by Professor Barbara Andersen, professor of psychology at Ohio State University. This is the basis of the whole approach to neuroscience: psychoneuroimmunology (an approach foreseen more than ten years earlier by Professor Claude Jasmin in his work at Villejuif). Professor Andersen set up a vast program of study in Ohio. It's interesting to highlight an amusing anecdote that reveals the resistance of the medical world in the face of new, nonmolecular (strictly nonchemical), therapeutic paths. Before the excellent results obtained by the 114 patients in this study (targeting the impact of mental and emotional training on the immune system's strength), Professor Andersen herself admitted, "We were so surprised with the findings about immunity that we repeated the tests over and over again." Yet the conclusions from the study are clear: the tools of mind-body medicine offered to the patients during the four months helped give them a measurable "immune vitality," superior to that of the control group (who even had a tendency to get worse).

Concentrating on Biorhythms Controls Asthma

Study led by Paul Lehrer at the psychophysiology laboratory at Robert Wood Johnson University in Piscataway, New Jersey. Details of the study are recounted on page 47 of this book as an introduction to Tool #1 (Delta Breathing).

Mental Stimulation Increases Muscle Strength

Study led by Guang Yue, physiologist at the Cleveland (Ohio) Clinic Foundation. A program of guided mental imagery, aimed at certain muscle groups, to visualize your body in action. The muscles can develop without any real movement.

Transcendental Meditation Lowers High Blood Pressure

Study led by Vernon Barnes, physiologist at the Medical College of Georgia in Augusta. The title speaks for itself, but the origin of the study is worth examining. Following the excellent article summarizing the study in *Science et Vie,* is a scientific case study aimed at the three major lines of inquiry: "In an attempt to understand the surprising powers of the psyche, the researchers now explore three means of mobilizing the latest advances in neurosciences. What better way to develop a new comprehension of life," comments Philippe Chambon. The three lines of inquiry are:

- a study of modified states of consciousness: how the brain focuses attention
- a study of cerebral plasticity: when the brain reconfigures to adapt
- a study of psychoneuroimmunology: a dialogue between the brain and the body

So are these new holistic standards of modern medicine innovative and revolutionary? Not in the least, emphasizes Esther Sternberg, chief of the Section on Neuroendocrine Immunology at the National Institutes of Health in Bethesda. Maryland. "In fact, it's an image both new and very ancient," she reminds us. "Before the sixteenth century and the thinking of Descartes, which reduced things to separate elements to understand them, Western thinking already had this holistic view. It's amazing to see this resurgence through the language of science." At the same time that knowledge about the mind-body relationship progresses, a new image of the human being takes shape as a holistic entity.

New ways of holistic thinking have been established in medical science. But keep in mind that holistic thinking guided human beings for over two thousand years (ever since Hippocrates). Often scorned (at times simply forgotten) during the past two centuries in the face of all-powerful allopathic medicine (indisputably "all-powerful" when it comes to acute illnesses and injuries, but more modestly so, even impotent, when dealing with viral, chronic, or degenerative diseases). This more respectful and more open, humanistic thinking has reappeared full force at the beginning of the twenty-first century to expand the spaces of dialogue and balance the discoveries of science. In the foreword to this book, Professor Claude Jasmin emphasizes the importance of this and its pertinence (he himself did scientific experiments on this with some of the biggest names in medical psychiatry and psychology).

We must integrate these new methods into our daily practice to create better, new, ethical, and credible tools for health. This is the spirit and hope of this book.

GLOSSARY

acid-alkaline balance: Indispensable balance in the body between acidifying substances and alkalizing substances. This balance helps the body avoid an excess of acidity, which causes microinflammations in tissues. These microinflammations can lead to many illnesses. Breathing and nutrition strongly influence it.

adrenal glands: Endocrine glands, one located at the upper tip of each of your kidneys; thus there are two adrenal glands in the body. They are pale yellow in color and weigh about 0.2 pound (5 g) each. The anatomical dissection of an adrenal gland shows that it is formed of two parts: the corticoadrenal (the cortical zone: external, where cortisol is secreted) and the medulloadrenal (the medullar area: internal, where adrenaline is produced).

adrenaline: Hormone produced by the central part of the adrenal glands that is secreted during times of stress. Adrenaline acts by prompting the cardiovascular, liver, and muscular systems to take action.

allopathic: System of medical practice that treats the symptoms of disease with agents that produce effects different from those produced by the disease. Also called conventional, modern, or Western medicine.

antioxidant: Substance that opposes the action of free radicals (unstable ionic elements, produced by oxidation, that, in excess, are harmful to tissues and accelerate the aging process).

autogenic training: A mind-body technique developed during the twentieth century by the German psychiatrist Johannes Heinrich Schultz. Autogenic training uses visualizations and deliberate self-willed sensations to help practitioners reach a state of profound physical, mental, and emotional relaxation. It is a major therapeutic tool for all illnesses associated with the pressures of daily life and excess stress.

autoimmune disease: Disease in which the immune system produces new antibodies in order to destroy its own tissues, as if they were microbial enemies.

carbohydrates: A generic term referring to all forms of sugar present in foods, from the most simple, like glucose, to the most complex, such as grains. Carbohydrates constitute the principal source of direct energy for the body, in combination with oxygen.

chemotherapy: Chemical treatments infused intravenously (or, now, in capsules) designed to treat certain types of cancer and degenerative illnesses.

degenerative disease: Disease characterized by the premature wearing out and then the progressive, inevitable degeneration of certain tissues and organs. Includes many types of cancer and certain kinds of diabetes, heart disease, hypertension, and dementia (nonsenile).

dopamine: A cerebral neurotransmitter that stimulates the nervous system's sense of satisfaction, reward, pleasure, optimism, etc.

draining: A practice consisting of stimulating the body's elimination functions (urination, defecation, perspiration) in order to accelerate the treatment and evacuation of internal and external wastes, such as toxic overload from pollution or medications.

enzyme: A substance synthesized by our organs, tissues, and cells that serves as a catalyst for the billions of biochemical reactions that make our bodies function and remain alive.

fascia: Tendinous tissue that connects, covers, holds, and supports the organs and muscular and osteotendinous structures of the body. The fascia is like the Ariadne's thread that keeps record of all our bodily tensions and overloads generated by excess stress and bad neuroemotional management.

fasting: Total deprivation of food for a specified amount of time (from a few days to a few weeks), meant to decontaminate and relax the body. Fasting often has a spiritual connotation, and is therefore often used in religious rites. Fasting can cause organ damage; it should be done under the supervision of a trusted health care practitioner and is not recommended for periods longer than 3 to 5 days.

free radicals: Highly reactive ionic substances produced naturally by the body under the influence of cellular oxidation. An excess of free radicals is damaging to a person's health, and contributes to premature aging of the tissues.

glycemic index (GI): A biological index applied to foods; it measures their impact on the production of insulin by the pancreas. The index ranges from 0 to 100. Proteins and fats have a low GI; grains and vegetables a moderate GI; simple sugars and alcohol a high GI.

immunity: A group of phenomena, coordinated by the immune system, that protect the body from microbial aggressors.

insulin: An essential hormone produced by the pancreas that ensures the stability of the blood sugar level.

lipids: All fats, including fatty acids and their derivatives (esters, aldehydes). These are the principal constituents of plasma membranes and adipose tissue. Lipids can be grouped into fatty acids, glycerides, phospholipids, and glycolipids. From a nutritional standpoint, lipids contribute the most calories (9.3 kcal/gram). Lipids prompt a wide variety of biological functions, principally the production of energy by beta oxidation and the formatting of hormonal messages. They play an essential role within the cell, constituting the structure of the lipid bilayer of cellular membranes.

lupus: A chronic cutaneous affliction that becomes serious when it takes the systemic form, thus affecting all the organs, the blood, and the bone marrow.

macrobiotic: An Eastern lifestyle based on the energetic laws (yin and yang) from Chinese (and Japanese) medicine and on the principles of Zen Buddhism. In Western societies most people are familiar with the nutritional aspects of the macrobiotic doctrine. This approach is at times dangerous because practitioners' understanding of its underpinnings is incomplete.

Metabolic Index: The overall index that classifies foods according to their impact on the pancreas (glycemic index), digestion (enzymatic index), and in small measure their energy contribution (caloric index).

mind-body: Referring to techniques with psychotherapeutic aims that employ the body and its functions (breathing, nutrition, exercise) in the healing process.

multiple sclerosis: A disease of the nervous system in which the myelin, a kind of sheath surrounding the nervous tissue, is altered and damaged. This progressive disease is characterized by attacks that vary in severity, followed by periods of remission that vary in duration.

neuron: A nerve cell that carries out the production and transmission of nervous impulses in the body. Neurons constitute the majority of brain and nerve matter and they are also found on the periphery of other organs, notably the intestines and the heart.

neurosis: An unresolved mental conflict, locked in the depths of the unconscious, that causes psychological blocks and inappropriate behaviors. The patient is conscious of the disturbance and of this disorder, unlike patients suffering from psychosis.

neurotransmitter: A hormonal substance that transmits nervous impulses in the brain and nervous system.

phytotherapy: A branch of medicine that consists of treatments with medicinal plants absorbed in various forms (decoction, infusion, aqueous or alcohol extracts, dried plant powders).

proteins: Substances made of amino acids and forming the major part of living tissues (notably muscles and organs); they are indispensable for tissue regeneration. Proteins are principally provided by foods derived from animals (meat, fish, eggs, dairy products).

psychiatry: A branch of medicine whose goal is to study and treat mental illnesses. Psychiatrists may use chemical medicine to relieve psychoemotional symptoms and ease neurological disorders.

psychoanalysis: A therapeutic cure developed by Sigmund Freud at the end of the nineteenth century. Psychoanalysis uses talking and free associating of ideas as a vehicle to unveil and resolve neuroses.

psychosis: A group of mental illnesses, which are usually serious (including schizophrenia, paranoia, and bipolar psychosis), that stem from biological troubles with the neurotransmitters. Different from neurosis in that patients are not (or are barely) conscious of their disorder.

psychotherapy: Talk therapy (within a patient/therapist dialogue context) that seeks to relieve psychoneuroemotional suffering. Contrary to psychoanalysis, psychotherapy's first-line treatment focuses on what takes place on the conscious level, rather than the unconscious level.

radiation therapy: A treatment using the effects of some types of ionizing rays on the tissues, with the goal of destroying certain kinds of cancers.

serotonin: A major cerebral hormone that acts as a mediator of information in the nervous system and brain. Serotonin is characteristic of states of balance and inner harmony.

sophrology: A series of physical and mental exercises (called dynamic relaxation) designed to produce a healthy, relaxed body and a calm, alert mind. Popular in French speaking countries where it is used in businesses, schools, sports, and hospitals.

synergy: A combination of several complementary treatments or techniques (medical or nonmedical) that act in concert to treat the same pathological manifestation more effectively.

trace element: A mineral or metal substance, present in very small quantities in the body and indispensable to its correct functioning. Trace elements are generally contributed through food.

tumor: Uncontrolled proliferation of cells. The growth of benign tumors is generally limited (even encapsulated), but in malignant tumors this is almost never the case. This uncontrolled growth leads to serious damage within the body because tumors possess their own inner life (with their own vascularization, breathing, and nutrition).

visualization: A mind-body technique using breathing, relaxation, and mental imagery training (guided imagery) for therapeutic purposes.

vitamin: A substance from the vast family of essential micronutrients, present in very small quantities in the body and indispensable to its correct functioning. Our body doesn't know how to synthesize these vitamins itself, so it must draw them out of food. If our diet or nutritional balance is poor, deficiencies occur. The weakening of the biological terrain then promotes the appearance of chronic or degenerative diseases.

yoga: A mind-body (and spiritual) technique that comes from the ancestral tradition of India. It uses physical postures, combined with breathing and meditative practices, to harmonize the physical and psychoemotional functions. There are various forms of yoga, from the most physical to the most spiritual. Several American and Canadian universities have created scientific programs to explore the biological effects of yoga. This has resulted in a more in-depth biological understanding of how to best put yoga to work as a healing modality.

INDEX

Page numbers in *italics* refer to illustrations.